Practical Workbook in Forensic Medicine and Toxicology

The Bengal Academy of Forensic Medicine

Practical Workbook in Forensic Medicine and Toxicology

As per the Competency Based Medical Education Curriculum (NMC)

Second Edition

Under the Aegis of

The Bengal Academy of Forensic Medicine

JAYPEE

JAYPEE BROTHERS MEDICAL PUBLISHERS

The Health Sciences Publisher

New Delhi | London

Jaypee Brothers Medical Publishers (P) Ltd

Headquarters
EMCA House
23/23-B, Ansari Road, Daryaganj
New Delhi 110 002, India
Landline: +91-11-23272143, +91-11-23272703
+91-11-23282021, +91-11-23245672
E-mail: jaypee@jaypeebrothers.com

Corporate Office
4838/24, Ansari Road, Daryaganj
New Delhi 110 002, India
Phone: +91-11-43574357
Fax: +91-11-43574314
E-mail: jaypee@jaypeebrothers.com

Overseas Office
J.P. Medical Ltd
83 Victoria Street, London
SW1H 0HW (UK)
Phone: +44 20 3170 8910
E-mail: info@jpmedpub.com

EU GPSR Authorised Representative
Logos Europe, 9 rue Nicolas Poussin
17000, La Rochelle, France
Phone: +33 (0) 6 67 93 73 78
E-mail: contact@logoseurope.eu

Website: www.jaypeebrothers.com
Website: www.jaypeedigital.com

Practical Workbook in Forensic Medicine and Toxicology

First Edition: 2019

Second Edition: 2023

Reprint: ***2026***

ISBN: 978-93-5465-897-6

Printed at: Sterling Graphics Pvt. Ltd. India.

Dedicated to

The Students

The Executive Committee of the BAFM 2025–2027

President
Parag Baran Pal

Vice-Presidents
Soumyajyoti Bandopadhyay
Sobhan Roy

Secretary
Arindam Chakrovarty

Joint Secretaries
Shibsankar Mahato
Rama Samaddar

Treasurer
Arijit Dey

Assistant Treasurer
Madhurima Mondal

Journal Editor
O Gambhir Singh

Journal Co-Editor
Rina Das

Executive Committee Members
Saurabh Chattopadhyay
Chandan Bandyopadhyay
Sujash Biswas
Abhishek Das
Sayan Biswas

Ex-officio Members
Biswajit Sukul
Somnath Das

Editorial Board

Preface to the Second Edition

This second edition of the *Practical Workbook in Forensic Medicine and Toxicology* mainly focuses on the competencies that has to be followed as per the new competency-based medical education (CBME) curriculum designed by NMC.

In this edition we have incorporated all the competencies that have to be followed in the syllabus of Forensic Medicine and Toxicology. It is preferable that the questions should cover the skills that is essential for a Indian medical graduates in this field. The colored picture and the format of the book will help the students for easy learning of this important subject.

Tapas Kumar Bose
Somnath Das

Preface to the First Edition

A problem-based workbook has been a long-felt need for the students pursuing the course of Forensic Medicine and Toxicology. In order to bring the uniformity in the teaching and training throughout the Medical Colleges of the State, the book will be of great help.

It is confidently believed that the book will furnish the students with the necessary number and variety of exercises essential to master the application of the subject. Most of the exercises come up with a guideline at the beginning to make it more convenient for the students to do the exercise.

All the exercise pages are carefully designed to eliminate distraction and to focus the pupils' full attention on the work in hand. Hopefully, the workbook will be a book to be preserved for the future use by the students in their forthcoming days of medicine practice.

Tapas Kumar Bose
Somnath Das

Name of the Student: ....

Name of the College: ....

Roll No. : ....

University Reg No. : ....

University Roll No. : ....

This book must be submitted during 2nd Professional MBBS practical examination. Student will not be allowed to appear on non-submission.

Contents

Instructions to Students

1. Punctually in attending practical classes should be maintained, as 80% attendance in practical is mandatory as per university rule.
2. Silence and discipline should be observed during practical work.
3. Clean apron should be worn before entering the practical hall.
4. Every student should bring the practical record book, a piece of clean linen, a measuring tape, stethoscope, torch, hammer and a hand lens and colored pencils.
5. Listen carefully to the instructions given by the teachers for the day's work.
6. After finishing the practical work, complete them in the record book, get the record checked by the teachers before next class.
7. Maintenance of cleanliness at the site of the practical work should be stressed.
8. All students must appear and clear all the item examinations on the stipulated date during the course.

Certificate of Completion

This is to certify that .... has submitted this practical notebook during 5th Semester Examination held in the month of......................................., 20.....................................

.... Demonstrator

.... Associate/Assistant Professor

.... Professor

University Reg No.: ....

University Roll No.: ....

This is to certify that .... has submitted this practical notebook during University Practical Examination held in the month of......................................., 20........................

.... Signature of Internal Examiner 2nd Professional Examination

.... Signature of External Examiner 2nd Professional Examination

CBME Curriculum

Teaching Methods and Hours

Phase	*Lectures (LGT)*	*Tutorials (SGT)*	*Practicals*	*Autopsy demo*	*AETCOM*	*Total*
2nd year	20 hours	5 hours	15 hours	5 hours	5 hours	50 hours
3rd year	35 hours	10 hours	20 hours	10 hours	0 hour	75 hours
Total	55 hours	15 hours	35 hours	15 hours	5 hours	125 hours

List of Competencies and SLOs to be Covered in Phase II MBBS

Sl. No. and competency codes	*Topics As per various competencies*	*Teaching/ learning methods*	*No. of hours*
1. Introduction to forensic medicine and toxicology			
FM1.1	Demonstrate knowledge of basics of forensic medicine like definitions of forensic medicine, clinical forensic medicine, forensic pathology, state medicine, legal medicine and medical jurisprudence.	LGT	1
FM1.2	Describe history of forensic medicine.		
2. Legal procedure			
FM1.3	Describe legal procedures including criminal procedure code, Indian Penal Code, Indian Evidence Act, civil and criminal cases, inquest, cognizable and non-cognizable offences, evidences.	LGT	1
FM1.4	Describe courts in India and their powers: Supreme court, high court, sessions court, magistrate's court, labor court, family court, executive magistrate court and juvenile justice board.		
FM1.5	Describe court procedures including issue of summons, conduct money, types of witnesses, recording of evidence, oath, affirmation, examination in chief, cross examination, re-examination and court questions, recording of evidence and conduct of doctor in witness box.	LGT	1
FM1.6	Describe offenses in court including perjury; court strictures vis-a-vis medical officer.		
FM2.29	Demonstrate respect to the directions of courts, while appearing as witness for recording of evidence under oath or affirmation, examination in chief, cross examination, re-examination and court questions, recording of evidence.	SGD	1
FM1.7	Describe dying declaration and dying deposition.	LGT	1
FM1.8	Describe the latest decisions/notifications/resolutions/circulars/standing orders related to medicolegal practice issued by courts/government.		
FM14.20	To record and certify dying declaration in a simulated/supervised environment.		
3. Death and its causes			
FM2.1	Define, describe and discuss death and its types including somatic/clinical/cellular, molecular and brain-death, cortical death and brainstem death.	LGT	1
FM2.2	Describe and discuss natural and unnatural deaths.		
FM2.5	Discuss moment of death, modes of death-coma, asphyxia and syncope.		
FM2.3	Describe and discuss issues related to sudden natural deaths.		
FM2.6	Discuss presumption of death and survivorship.	LGT	1
FM2.7	Describe and discuss suspended animation.		
FM2.4	Describe salient features of the organ transplantation and the Human Organ Transplant (Amendment) Act 2011 and discuss ethical issues regarding organ donation.	LGT	1

Sl. No. and competency codes	Topics As per various competencies	Teaching/ learning methods	No. of hours
FM1.10	Select appropriate cause of death in a particular scenario by referring ICD 10 code.	SGT	1
FM1.11	Write a correct cause of death certificate as per ICD 10 document.		
4. Postmortem changes			
FM2.8	Describe and discuss postmortem changes including signs of death, cooling of body, postmortem lividity, rigor mortis, cadaveric spasm, cold stiffening and heat stiffening.	LGT	2
FM2.9	Describe putrefaction, mummification, adipocere and maceration.	LGT	1
FM2.10	Discuss estimation of time since death.		
5. Autopsy procedure			
FM2.12	Describe the legal requirements to conduct postmortem examination and procedures to conduct medicolegal postmortem examination.	LGT	2
FM2.11	Describe and discuss autopsy procedures including postmortem examination, different types of autopsies, aims and objectives of postmortem examination.		
FM2.14	Describe and discuss examination of clothing, preservation of viscera on postmortem examination for chemical analysis and other medicolegal purposes, postmortem artefacts.	LGT	1
FM2.13	Describe and discuss obscure autopsy.		
FM2.17	Describe and discuss exhumation.		
6. Identification			
FM3.1	Define and describe Corpus Delicti, establishment of identity of living persons including race, sex, religion, complexion, stature, age determination using morphology, teeth-eruption, decay, bitemarks, bones-ossification centers, medicolegal aspects of age.	LGT	4
FM14.9	Demonstrate examination of and present an opinion after examination of skeletal remains in a simulated/supervised environment.	SGT Practical	4
FM14.4	Conduct and prepare report of estimation of age of a person for medicolegal and other purposes and prepare medicolegal report in a simulated/supervised environment.		
FM3.2	Describe and discuss identification of criminals, unknown persons, dead bodies from the remains—hairs, fibers, teeth, anthropometry, dactylography, footprints, scars, tattoos, poroscopy and superimposition.	Practical Demo	10
FM14.6	Demonstrate and interpret medicolegal aspects from examination of hair (human and animal) fiber, semen and other biological fluids.		
7. Mechanical injuries			
FM3.3	Define, describe and classify different types of mechanical injuries, abrasion, bruise, laceration, stabwound, incised wound, chop wound, defense wound, self-inflicted/fabricated wounds and their medicolegal aspects.	LGT	3
FM3.6	Describe healing of injury and fracture of bones with its medicolegal importance.		
FM3.7	Describe factors influencing infliction of injuries and healing, examination and certification of wounds and wound as a cause of death: Primary and secondary.	SGT Practical	1
FM14.1	Examine and prepare medicolegal report of an injured person with different etiologies in a simulated/supervised environment.	SGT	1
FM3.4	Mechanical injuries and wounds: Define injury, assault and hurt. Describe IPC pertaining to injuries accidental, suicidal and homicidal injuries.	LGT	2
FM3.5	Describe simple, grievous and dangerous injuries. Describe antemortem and postmortem injuries.		
FM3.8	Mechanical injuries and wounds: Describe and discuss different types of weapons including dangerous weapons and their examination.	SGT Practical	2
FM14.11	To identify and describe weapons of medicolegal importance which are commonly used, e.g., lathi, knife, kripan, axe, gandasa, gupti, farsha, dagger, bhalla, razor and stick. Able to prepare report of the weapons brought by police and to give opinion regarding injuries present on the person as described in injury report/PM report so as to connect weapon with the injuries. (Prepare injury report/PM report must be provided to connect the weapon with the injuries).		

Sl. No. and competency codes	Topics As per various competencies	Teaching/ learning methods	No. of hours
8. Firearm injuries			
FM3.9	Describe different types of firearms including structure and components. Along with description of ammunition propellant charge and mechanism of fire-arms, different types of cartridges and bullets and various terminology in relation to firearm–caliber, range, choking.	LGT	2
FM3.10	Describe and discuss wound ballistics-different types of firearm injuries, blast injuries and their interpretation, preservation and dispatch of trace evidence in cases of firearm and blast injuries, various tests related to confirmation of use of firearms.		
FM14.12	Describe the contents and structure of bullet and cartridges used and to provide medicolegal interpretation from these.		
9. Regional injuries			
FM3.11	Describe and discuss regional injuries to head (scalp wounds, fracture skull, intracranial hemorrhages, coup and contrecoup injuries), neck, chest, abdomen, limbs, genital organ, spinal cord and skeleton.	LGT	2
FM3.12	Regional injuries describe and discuss injuries related to fall from height and vehicular injuries–primary and secondary impact, secondary injuries, crush syndrome, railway spine.		
10. Mechanical asphyxia			
FM2.20	Define, classify and describe asphyxia and medicolegal interpretation of postmortem findings in asphyxial deaths.	LGT	2
FM2.21	Describe and discuss different types of hanging and strangulation including clinical findings, causes of death, postmortem findings and medicolegal aspects of death due to hanging and strangulation including examination, preservation and dispatch of ligature material.	Autopsy Demo	1
FM2.22	Describe and discuss pathophysiology, clinical features, postmortem findings and medicolegal aspects of traumatic asphyxia, obstruction of nose and mouth, suffocation and sexual asphyxia.	LGT	1
FM2.23	Describe and discuss types, pathophysiology, clinical features, postmortem findings and medicolegal aspects of drowning, diatom test and, gettler test.	LGT Autopsy Demo	1 1
11. Medical law and ethics			
FM4.1	Describe medical ethics and explain its historical emergence.	LGT	1
FM4.2	Describe the Code of Medical Ethics 2002 conduct, etiquette and ethics in medical practice.		
FM4.3	And unethical practices and the dichotomy describe the functions and role of medical.		
FM4.4	Council of India and State Medical Councils. Describe the Indian Medical Register.		
FM4.5	Rights/privileges of a medical practitioner, penal erasure, infamous conduct, disciplinary Committee, disciplinary procedures, warning notice and penal erasure.		
FM4.6	Describe the laws in relation to medical practice and the duties of a medical practitioner towards patients and society.		
FM4.28	Demonstrate respect to laws relating to medical practice and ethical code of conduct prescribed by Medical Council of India and rules and regulations prescribed by it from time to time.		
FM4.24	Enumerate rights, privileges and duties of a Registered Medical Practitioner. Discuss doctor-patient relationship: professional secrecy and privileged communication.	AETCOM	1
FM4.19	Define consent. Describe different types of consent and ingredients of informed consent. Describe the rules of consent and importance of consent in relation to age, emergency situation, mental illness and alcohol intoxication.	AETCOM	1
FM4.20	Describe therapeutic privilege, malingering, therapeutic misadventure, professional secrecy, human experimentation.	SGT	1
FM4.21	Describe products liability and medical indemnity insurance.		
FM4.17	Describe and discuss ethical principles: Respect for autonomy, non-malfeasance, beneficence and justice.	LGT	1

Sl. No. and competency codes	*Topics As per various competencies*	*Teaching/ learning methods*	*No. of hours*
FM4.18	Describe and discuss medical negligence including civil and criminal negligence, contributory negligence, corporate negligence, vicarious liability, Res Ipsa Loquitor, prevention of medical negligence and defenses in medical negligence litigations.		
FM4.8	Describe the Consumer Protection Act 1986 (Medical Indemnity Insurance, Civil Litigations and Compensations), Workman's Compensation Act and ESI Act.	AETCOM	1
FM4.11	Describe and discuss euthanasia.	LGT	1
FM4.22 FM4.23	Explain Oath—Hippocrates, Charaka and Sushruta and procedure for administration of oath.		
FM4.16	Describe the modified declaration of Geneva and its relevance.	AETCOM	1
FM4.27	Describe and discuss bioethics.	AETCOM	1
FM4.25	Describe and discuss ethical guidelines for biomedical research on human subjects and animals clinical research and ethics. Discuss human experimentation including clinical trials.		
12. Thermal injuries			
FM2.24	Describe the clinical features, postmortem finding and medicolegal aspects of injuries due to physical agents like heat (heat-hyper-pyrexia, heat stroke, sun stroke, heat exhaustion/ prostration, heat cramps (miner's cramp) or cold (systemic localized) hypothermia, frostbite, trench foot, immersion foot.	LGT	2
FM2.25	Describe types of injuries, clinical features, pathophysiology, postmortem findings and medicolegal aspects in cases of burns, scalds, lightening, electrocution and radiations.		
13. Documentation certifications			
FM1.9	Describe the importance of documentation in medical practice in regard to medicolegal examinations, medical certificates and medico legal reports especially—maintenance of patient case records, discharge summary, prescribed registers to be maintained in health centers.	SGT	1
	1. Documents for estimation of age by physical, dental and radiological examination and issuance of certificate.	AETCOM	1
	2. Maintenance of medicolegal register like accident register.	Practical	4
	3. Documents of issuance of wound certificate.	SGT	1
	4. Documents of issuance of sickness and fitness certificate.	Practical	2
	5. Documents for issuance of death certificate.		
	6. Documents of medical certification of cause of death - Form number 4 and 4A.	SGT	1
	7. Documents of issuance of drunkenness certificate.	SGT	1
14. Impotence sterility ART			
FM3.18	Describe anatomy of male and female genitalia, hymen and its types. Discuss the medicolegal importance of hymen. Define virginity, defloration, legitimacy, medicolegal importance.	LGT	3
FM3.22	Define and discuss impotence, sterility, frigidity, sexual dysfunction, premature ejaculation Discuss the causes of impotence and sterility in male and female.		
FM3.23	Discuss sterilization of male and female, artificial insemination, test tube baby, surrogate mother, hormonal replacement therapy with respect to appropriate national and state laws.		
FM3.20	Discuss disputed paternity and maternity.		
15. Virginity pregnancy delivery			
FM3.19	Discuss the medicolegal aspects of pregnancy and delivery, signs of pregnancy, precipitate labor superfetation, superfecundation and signs of recent and remote delivery in living and dead.	LGT	2
FM3.21	Discuss preconception and prenatal diagnostic techniques (PC and PNDT) - Prohibition of Sex Selection Act 2003 and Domestic Violence Act 2005.		
FM3.24	Discuss the relative importance of surgical methods of contraception (vasectomy and tubectomy) as methods of contraception in the National Family Planning Programme.		

Sl. No. and competency codes	*Topics As per various competencies*	*Teaching/ learning methods*	*No. of hours*
16. Abortion MTP			
FM3.27	Define, classify and discuss abortion, methods of procuring MTP and criminal abortion and complication of abortion. MTP Act 1971.	LGT	2
FM3.28	Describe evidences of abortion—living and dead, duties of doctor in cases of abortion, investigations of death due to criminal abortion.		
17. Live birth still birth infanticide			
FM2.28	Describe and discuss signs of intrauterine death, signs of live birth, viability of fetus, age determination of fetus, DOAP session of ossification centers, hydrostatic test, sudden infants death syndrome and Munchausen's syndrome by proxy.	LGT	2
FM2.27	Define and discuss infanticide, feticide and stillbirth.		
FM3.29	Describe and discuss child abuse and battered baby syndrome.		
FM14.13	To estimate the age of fetus by postmortem examination.	Practical	2
18. Torture			
FM3.30	Describe and discuss issues relating to torture, identification of injuries caused by torture and its sequelae, management of torture survivors.	LGT	1
FM3.31	Torture and human rights describe and discuss guidelines and protocols of national human rights commission regarding torture.		
19. Sexual offences			
FM3.13	Describe different types of sexual offences. Describe various sections of IPC regarding rape including definition of rape (Section 375 IPC), Punishment for Rape (Section 376 IPC) and recent amendments notified till date.	LGT	1
FM3.14	Describe and discuss the examination of the victim of an alleged case of rape, and the preparation of report, framing the opinion and preservation and dispatch of trace evidences in such cases.	LGT	1
FM3.15	Describe and discuss examination of accused and victim of sodomy, preparation of report, framing of opinion, preservation and dispatch of trace evidences in such cases.	LGT	1
FM3.16	Describe and discuss adultery and unnatural sexual offence sodomy, incest, lesbianism, buccal coitus, bestiality, indecent assault and preparation of report, framing the opinion and preservation and dispatch of trace evidences in such cases.	LGT	1
FM3.17	Describe and discuss the sexual perversions fetishism, transvestism, voyeurism, sadism, necrophagia, masochism, exhibitionism, frotteurim necrophilia.		
FM14.14	To examine and prepare report of an alleged accused in rape/unnatural sexual offence in a simulated/supervised environment.	Practical	3
FM14.15	To examine and prepare medicolegal report of a victim of sexual offence/unnatural sexual offence in a simulated/supervised environment.		
20. Forensic serology			
FM6.1	Describe different types of specimen and tissues to be collected both in the living and dead: Body fluids (blood, urine, semen, feces saliva), skin, nails, tooth pulp, vaginal smear, viscera, skull, specimen for histopathological examination, blood grouping, HLA typing and DNA fingerprinting. Describe Locard's exchange principle.	LGT	1
FM6.2	Describe the methods of sample collection, preservation, labelling, dispatch, and interpretation of reports.	SGT	1
FM6.3	Demonstrate professionalism while sending the biological or trace evidences to forensic science laboratory, specifying the required tests to be carried out, objectives of preservation of evidences sent for examination, personal discussions on interpretation of findings.	Practical	4
FM14.7	Demonstrate and identify that a particular stain is blood and identify the species of its origin.		
FM14.8	Demonstrate the correct technique to perform and identify ABO and RH blood group of a person		
FM14.21	To collect, preserve, seal and dispatch exhibits for DNA-finger printing using various formats of different laboratories.		

Sl. No. and competency codes	*Topics As per various competencies*	*Teaching/ learning methods*	*No. of hours*
21. Recent advances and FSL			
FM7.1	Enumerate the indications and describe the principles and appropriate use for: • DNA profiling—facial reconstruction. • Polygraph (lie detector)—narcoanalysis, brain mapping, digital autopsy, virtual autopsy, imaging technologies.	LGT	1
FM8.10	Describe the general principles of analytical toxicology and give a brief description of analytical methods available for toxicological analysis: Chromatography—thin layer chromatography, gas chromatography, liquid chromatography and atomic absorption spectroscopy.	LGT	1
22. Forensic psychiatry			
FM5.1	Classify common mental illnesses including post-traumatic stress disorder (PTSD).	LGT	1
FM5.2	Define, classify and describe delusions, hallucinations, illusion, lucid interval and obsessions with exemplification.		
FM5.3	Describe civil and criminal responsibilities of a mentally ill person.	LGT	1
FM5.4	Differentiate between true insanity from feigned insanity.		
FM5.5	Describe and discuss delirium tremens.	LGT	1
FM5.6	Describe the Indian Mental Health Act, 1987 with special reference to admission, care and discharge of a mentally ill person.		
23. General toxicology			
FM8.1	Describe the history of toxicology.	LGT	1
FM8.2	Define the terms toxicology, forensic toxicology, clinical toxicology and poison.		
FM8.3	Describe the various types of poisons, toxicokinetics and toxicodynamics and diagnosis of poisoning in living and dead.		
FM8.4	Describe the Laws in relations to poisons including NDPS Act, Medicolegal aspects of poisons. S. 85 IPC, S. 86 IPC, S. 274 IPC, S. 284 IPC, S. 299 IPC, S. 300 IPC, S. 304 (A) IPC, S. 375 IPC, S. 324 IPC, S. 325 IPC, S. 326 IPC, S. 326A IPC, S. 326B IPC, S. 328 IPC S. 357C CrPC S. 185 IMV Act, S. 203 IMV Act, S. 204 IMV Act.	LGT	1
FM8.5	Describe medicolegal autopsy in cases of poisoning including preservation and dispatch of viscera for chemical analysis.		
FM8.6	Describe the general symptoms, principles of diagnosis and management of common poisons encountered in India.		
FM8.7	Describe simple bedside clinic tests to detect poison/drug in a patient's body fluids.	LGT	1
FM8.8	Describe basic methodologies in treatment of poisoning: Decontamination, supportive therapy, antidote therapy, procedures of enhanced elimination.		
FM8.9	Describe the procedure of intimation of suspicious cases or actual cases of foul play to the police, maintenance of records, preservation and dispatch of relevant samples for laboratory analysis.	SGT	1
24. Corrosives			
FM9.1	Describe general principles and basic methodologies in treatment of poisoning: Decontamination, supportive therapy, antidote therapy, procedures of enhanced elimination with regard to: Caustics inorganic—sulphuric, nitric, and hydrochloric acids; organic—carboloic acid (phenol), oxalic and acetylsalicylic acids.	LGT Practical	
25. Inorganic irritants			
FM9.2	Describe general principles and basic methodologies in treatment of poisoning: Decontamination, supportive therapy, antidote therapy, procedures of enhanced elimination with regard to phosphorus, iodine, barium.	LGT Practical	1 1
26. Heavy metals			
FM9.3	Describe general principles and basic methodologies in treatment of poisoning: Decontamination, supportive therapy, antidote therapy, procedures of enhanced elimination with regard to arsenic, lead, mercury, copper, iron, cadmium and thallium.	LGT Practical	2 2

Sl. No. and competency codes	*Topics As per various competencies*	*Teaching/ learning methods*	*No. of hours*
27. Alcohol			
FM9.4	Describe general principles and basic methodologies in treatment of poisoning: Decontamination, supportive therapy, antidote therapy, procedures of enhanced elimination with regard to ethanol, methanol, ethylene glycol.	LGT	2
FM14.16	To examine and prepare medicolegal report of drunk person in a simulated/supervised environment	SGT Practical	1 1
28. Insecticides pesticides			
FM9.5	Describe general principles and basic methodologies in treatment of poisoning: Decontamination, supportive therapy, antidote therapy, procedures of enhanced elimination with regard to organophosphates, carbamates, organochlorines, pyrethroids, paraquat, aluminium and zinc phosphide.	LGT Practical Autopsy Demo	2 1 1
29. FM9.6	Describe general principles and basic methodologies in treatment of poisoning: Decontamination, supportive therapy, antidote therapy, procedures of enhanced elimination with regard to ammonia, carbon monoxide, hydrogen cyanide and derivatives, methyl isocyanate, tear (riot control) gases.	LGT	1
30. FM12.1	Describe features and management of abuse/poisoning with following chemicals: Tobacco, cannabis, amphetamines, cocaine, hallucinogens, designer drugs and solvent.	LGT	1
31. FM11.1	Describe features and management of snake bite, scorpion sting, bee and wasp sting and spider bite	LGT Practical	2 1
32. FM10.1	Describe general principles and basic methodologies in treatment of poisoning: Decontamination, supportive therapy, antidote therapy, procedures of enhanced elimination with regard to: • **Antipyretics**—paracetamol, salicylates • **Anti-infectives** (common antibiotics—an overview) • **Neuropsychotoxicology**—barbiturates, benzodiazepines, phenytoin, lithium, haloperidol, neuroleptics, tricyclics • **Narcotic**—analgesics, anaesthetics, and muscle relaxants • **Cardiovascular toxicology**—cardiotoxic plants—oleander, nerium odorum, aconite, digitalis • **Gastrointestinal** and endocrinal drugs—insulin.	LGT LGT	1 1
33. FM13.1	Describe toxic pollution of environment, its medicolegal aspects and toxic hazards of occupation and industry.	LGT	1
34. FM14.5	Conduct and prepare postmortem examination report of varied etiologies (at least 15) in a simulated/supervised environment.	Autopsy Demo	12
35. FM14.10	Demonstrate ability to identify and prepare medicolegal inference from specimens obtained from various types of injuries, e.g., contusion, abrasion, laceration, firearm wounds, burns, head injury and fracture of bone.		
36. Investigation of anesthetic, operative deaths			
FM2.19	Describe and discuss special protocols for conduction of autopsy and for collection, preservation and dispatch of related material evidences: • Explain the significance of autopsy in operative deaths • Describe the procedure of autopsy in operative deaths • Describe the procedure of preservation and dispatch of evidentiary material for investigation in deaths associated with anesthesia and surgery.	SDL	1
37. Examination of mutilated bodies or fragments, charred bones and bundle of bones			
FM2.16	Describe and discuss examination of mutilated bodies or fragments, charred bones and bundle of bones: • Describe the procedure of examination of mutilated bodies/fragments • Describe the procedure of examination of skeletal remains (including charred bones).	SGD	1
FM14.9	Demonstrate examination of and present an opinion after examination of skeletal remains in a simulated/supervised environment: • Enumerate the objectives of skeletal remains examination • Demonstrate the procedure of examination of skeletal remains in a simulated/supervised environment • Draft a medicolegal report and opinion after examination of skeletal remains.	SGD	1

Sl. No. and competency codes	*Topics As per various competencies*	*Teaching/ learning methods*	*No. of hours*
38. Crime Scene Investigation			
FM2.18	Describe and discuss the objectives of crime scene visit, the duties and responsibilities of doctors on crime scene and the reconstruction of sequence of events after crime scene investigation: • Enumerate the objectives of crime scene visit by an autopsy surgeon • Describe the procedure of examination of crime scene and preservation of evidentiary material • Explain the reconstruction of a case after the crime scene visit.	SGD	1
39. FM2.31	Demonstrate ability to work in a team for conduction of medicolegal autopsies in cases of death following alleged medical negligence, dowry death, death in custody or following violation of human rights as per National Human Rights Commission Guidelines on exhumation: • Demonstrate the benefit of team work in a medicolegal autopsy of alleged medical negligence • Demonstrate the benefit of team work in a medicolegal autopsy of alleged dowry death • **2.31.3:** Demonstrate the benefit of team work in a medicolegal autopsy of alleged custodial death • **2.31.4:** Demonstrate the benefit of team work in a medicolegal autopsy of death due to violation of human rights • **2.31.5:** Demonstrate the benefit of team work in exhumation.	SDL	1
40. FM2.15	Describe special protocols for conduction of medicolegal autopsies in cases of death in custody or following violation of human rights as per National Human Rights Commission Guidelines • **2.15.1:** Describe the National Human Rights Commission guidelines for conduction of medicolegal autopsy in cases of death in custody or violation of human rights.	SGD	1
41. FM2.32	Demonstrate ability to exchange information by verbal or nonverbal communication to the peers, family members, law enforcing agency and judiciary • Demonstrate the skills of communication by a doctor with the peers • Demonstrate the skills of communication by a doctor with the patient's family members in MLC works at casualty • Demonstrate the skills of communication by a doctor with the deceased family members during medicolegal autopsy • Demonstrate the skills of communication by a doctor with the law enforcing agency/judiciary in medicolegal practices.		
42. FM2.35	Demonstrate professionalism while conducting autopsy in medicolegal situations, interpretation of findings and making inference/opinion, collection, preservation and dispatch of biological or trace evidences. **2.35.1:** Demonstrate the professionalism of a doctor during conduction of medicolegal autopsies (such as interaction with investigating officer/relatives of deceased, receiving inquest form, maintaining confidentiality, etc.). • Demonstrate the professionalism in preservation and dispatching evidentiary materials to FSL (such as proper method of preservation and dispatch of materials with necessary forms and maintaining confidentiality). • Demonstrate the professionalism in preservation and dispatching evidentiary materials to histopathology and microbiology investigations (such as proper method of preservation and dispatch of materials with necessary forms and maintaining confidentiality). **2.35.4:** Demonstrate the professionalism while giving opinion in medicolegal cases (such as honesty with unbiased inferences).	SGD	2

National Medical Commission (Undergraduate Medical Education Board)

In view of the court orders in WP(c) No. 7284 of 2021 titled Ms S Sushma and Anr. Vs The Commissioner of Police and Ors., the expert committee formed by Undergraduate Medical Education Board recommended modifications in the competencies (CBME) of Forensic Medicine subject Nos. **FM 3.16, FM 3.13, FM 3.17, FM 3.18** and competencies of psychiatric subject Nos. **PS 13.1 to 13.7** as follows:

Sl. No.	*Existing competency*	*Modified competency*
		Forensic medicine competency
1.	**FM3.16:** Describe and discuss adultery and unnatural sexual offences-sodomy, incest, lesbianism, buccal coitus, bestiality, indecent assault and preparation of report, framing the opinion and preservation and despatch of trace evidences in such cases.	**FM 3.16:** • Describe and discuss informed consent in sexual intercourse. • Describe and discuss histories of gender and sexuality-based (sexual orientation) identities and rights in India. • Describe history of decriminalization of 'adultery' and consensual adult homosexual sexual behavior. • Describe sexual offences with its medicolegal significance: – Forced/non-consensual penetrative anal sex – Forced/non-consensual oral sex – Sexual acts with animals/bestiality/zoophilia – Forced/non-consensual insertion of fingers or objects – Forced/non-consensual touching or groping or disrobing ('indecent assault').
2.	**FM3.13:** Describe different types of sexual offences. Describe various sections of IPC regarding rape including definition of rape (Section 375 IPC), Punishment for Rape (Section 376 IPC) and recent amendments notified till date.	**FM3.13:** • Describe various sections of IPC and CrPC related to definition of rape and sexual assault, medical examination of rape victim and accused of rape, police information by the doctors and medical care with recent amendments notified till date (i.e., Section 375 IPC, 166 B IPC, 357 C and 164 A, 53 A of CrPC). • Describe the relevant provisions of POCSO act related to medical examination, emergency medical care and police information.
3.	**FM3.17:** Describe and discuss the sexual perversions fetishism, transvestism, voyeurism, sadism, necrophagia, masochism, exhibitionism, frotteurism, necrophilia.	**FM3.17:** • Describe the difference between paraphilia and paraphilic disorder. Describe paraphilic disorder as per as per the latest guidelines of DSM and ICD and describe medico-legal implications of paraphilic disorder by referring scientific literature and legal justification (if any). • Describe and discuss the various paraphilias in the context of informed consent during any sexual interaction.
4.	**FM3.18:** Describe anatomy of male and female genitalia, hymen and its types. Discuss the medicolegal importance of hymen. Define virginity, defloration, legitimacy and its medicolegal importance.	**FM3.18:** • Describe legitimacy and its medicolegal importance. • Describe and discuss how 'signs' of virginity (so called 'virginity test', including finger tests on female genitalia) are unscientific, inhuman and discriminatory. • Describe and discuss how to appraise the courts about unscientific basis of these tests if court orders it.
5.	**FM14.14:** To examine and prepare report of an alleged accused in rape/ unnatural sexual offence in a simulated/supervised environment.	**FM14.14:** • To examine and prepare report on an alleged accused person in cases of various sexual offences in a simulated/supervised environment. • Demonstrate an understanding of framing the opinion, preservation and despatch of trace evidences in such cases. • Describe and discuss personal opinions and their impact on such examinations and the need for objectivity/neutrality to avoid prejudice influencing the case.

Sl. No.	Existing competency	Modified competency
6.	**FM14.15:** To examine and prepare medicolegal report of a victim of sexual offence/ unnatural sexual offence in a simulated/supervised environment.	**FM 14.15:** • To examine and prepare medicolegal report on an alleged victim of various sexual offences in a simulated/supervised environment. (Guidelines and Protocols of Medico Legal Care for Survivors Victims of Sexual Violence. Ministry of Health and Family Welfare, GOI-with latest modifications if any). • Demonstrate an understanding of framing the opinion and preservation and despatch of trace evidences in such cases. • Describe and discuss sympathetic/empathetic examination and interview of victims of sexual assault, including presence of trusted adult figure in cases of minor victims.
		Psychiatry competency
7.	**Topic name:** Psychosexual and gender identity disorders (Vol II **Page 210**).	**Topic name:** • Human sexuality • Gender incongruence or gender dysphoria • Gender nonconformity • Differences of sex development (DSD) or intersex • Paraphilia and paraphilic disorders • Sexual dysfunctions
8.	**PS13.1:** Enumerate and describe the magnitude and etiology of psychosexual and gender identity disorders. **PS13.2:** Enumerate, elicit, describe and document clinical features in patients with magnitude and etiology of psychosexual and gender identity disorders. **PS13.3:** Enumerate and describe the indications and interpret laboratory and other tests used in psychosexual and gender identity disorders. **PS13.4:** Describe the treatment of psychosexual and gender identity disorders including behavioral, psychosocial and pharmacologic therapy. **PS13.5:** Demonstrate family education in a patient with psychosexual and gender identity disorders in a simulated environment.	**PS13.1:** • Demonstrate an understanding of difference between sex and gender/biological and social construction of personhood. • Demonstrate an understanding of gender identity. • Demonstrate an understanding of transgender, gender nonconformity, and other gender diverse identities. • Demonstrate an understanding of sexual/sexuality identity, sexual orientation, sexual desire. • Demonstrate an understanding of the wide variety of sexual orientations and desires. • Describe and demonstrate an understanding of the differences in sex development in individuals who don't fit into the biological binary of male or female. • Demonstrate an understanding of common myths and misconceptions about LGBTQIA + identities like Hijra, Intersex. • Demonstrate an attitude of openness and respect for all genders and sexualities. • Demonstrate an understanding of common psychosocial stressor faced by members of LGBTQIA+ communities in India. • Demonstrate knowledge about basic tenets of LGBTQIA+ affirmative counseling. **PS13.2:** Demonstrate the ability to assess the gender identity of an individual and distress caused (if any) due to the individual's own gender identity in a simulated environment. **PS13.3:** Describe and understand how to discuss sexual orientation, sexuality identity, gender identity, as well as intersex identity (differences in sex development) as part of routine history taking. **PS13.4:** • Demonstrate in simulated environment the ability to educate and counsel individuals or family members about intersex variations, sexual orientations, sexuality identities, gender incongruence, gender dysphoria, and gender identities. • Demonstrate knowledge that conversion therapy practices for sexual orientation or gender identity or on people with intersex variations are unethical. **PS13.5:** • Describe differences between gender incongruence and gender dysphoria. • Describe and demonstrate an understanding of the biological and gender binaries, rejection of gender binary, gender nonconforming, gender nonbinary, androgynoiis, and other identities.

Sl. No.	*Existing competency*	*Modified competency*
	PS13.6: Enumerate and describe the pharmacologic basis and side effects of drugs used in psychosexual and gender identity disorders.	**PS13.6:** • Describe and discuss gender dysphoria. • Enumerate criteria to diagnose gender dysphoria according to the latest psychiatric classifications (refer to WPATH guidelines) and when to refer an individual to a mental health professional.
	PS13.7: Enumerate the appropriate conditions for specialist referral.	**PS13.7:** • Demonstrate in the simulated environment the ability to educate an individual and family members that gender incongruence by itself is not a disorder and does not require clinical intervention. • Discuss situations where there is a role for mental health support in gender dysphoria, i.e., discussing with faintly, deciding on hormonal treatments or sex reassignment surgery (gender affirming care or gender affirmative therapies or gender confirmation surgery). • Demonstrate in simulated environment the ability to educate and counsel individual and family members about various types of sexual orientation being normal.
		PS13.8: • Demonstrate in simulated environment the ability to educate an individual and family members that the gender of an individual can be different than the sex assigned at birth and also educate about the difference between sex and gender of an individual. • Demonstrate the ability to assess gender incongruence in an individual with intersex variations due to their gender identity. • Demonstrate knowledge and ability to educate family members that unnecessary medical interventions on individual with intersex variations are unethical.
		PS13.9: • Describe the difference between paraphilia and paraphilic disorder. • Describe different paraphilias. • Describe and discuss the importance of informed consent during any sexual interaction. • Describe and discuss impact of personal opinions on working with people who express paraphilias.
		PS13.10: Describe the prevalence and etiology of paraphilic disorders.
		PS13.11: Enumerate criteria for the diagnosis (diagnostic criteria) of paraphilic disorders according to the latest psychiatric classification.
		PS13.12: Demonstrate in the simulated environment the ability to educate the individual/ family members that paraphilia in itself is not a disease and may not require clinical intervention.
		PS13.13: Enumerate the reasons for specialist referrals for any of the cases.
		PS13.14: Describe the stages and differences in the human sexual cycle.
		PS13.15: Enumerate the diagnostic criteria of various sexual dysfunctions corresponding to the stage of the human sexual cycle.
		PS13.16: Describe the management (till the level of MBBS graduate domain) and reasons for specialist referral in cases of sexual dysfunction.

DACTYLOGRAPHY
(Study of Fingerprints)

Fingerprint (Definition):

Importance:

Classification of Fingerprint Patterns

Identify the following fingerprint patterns and mention their types and average distribution:

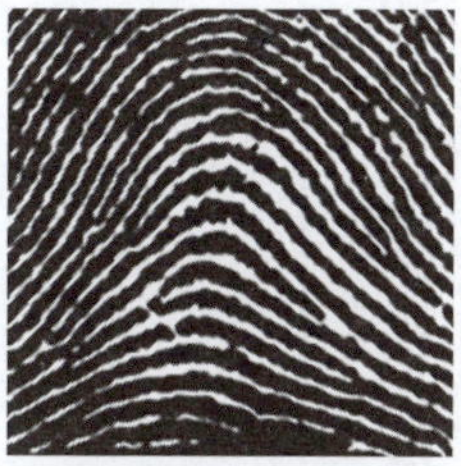

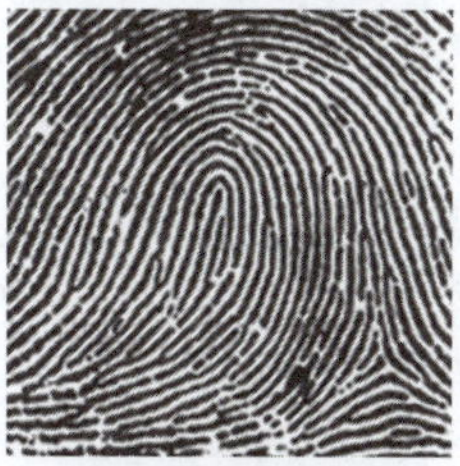

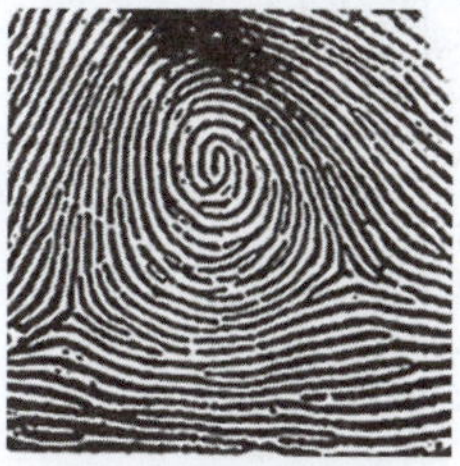

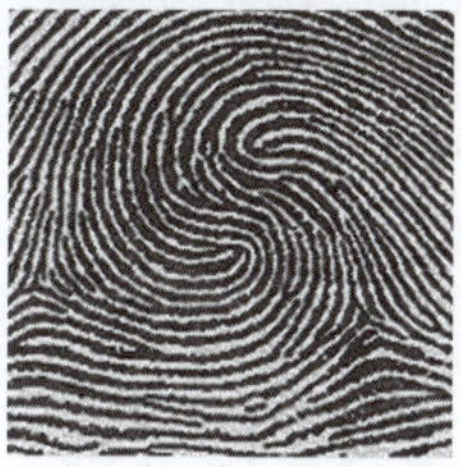

DACTYLOGRAPHY

Put the Impression of Your Own Fingerprint and Identify the Type

FINGERPRINT RECORD (Left)

Thumb		Index		Middle		Ring		Little	
Plain	*Rolled*	*Plain*	*Rolled*	*Plain*	*Rolled*	*Plain*	*Rolled*	*Plain*	*Rolled*

....

FINGERPRINT RECORD (Right)

Thumb		Index		Middle		Ring		Little	
Plain	*Rolled*	*Plain*	*Rolled*	*Plain*	*Rolled*	*Plain*	*Rolled*	*Plain*	*Rolled*

....

Signature of Student

EXAMINATION OF BONES (SEX)

Skull:

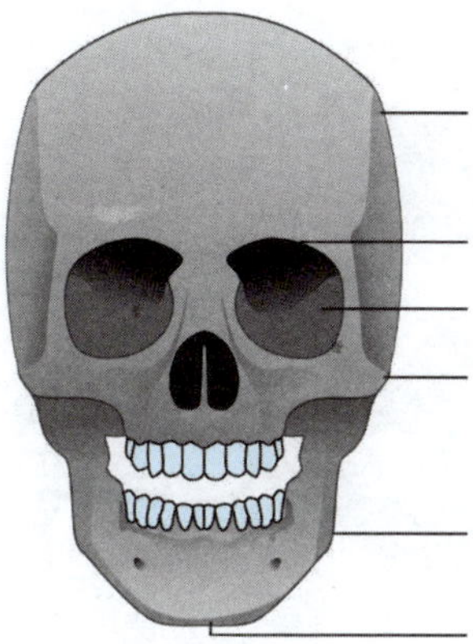

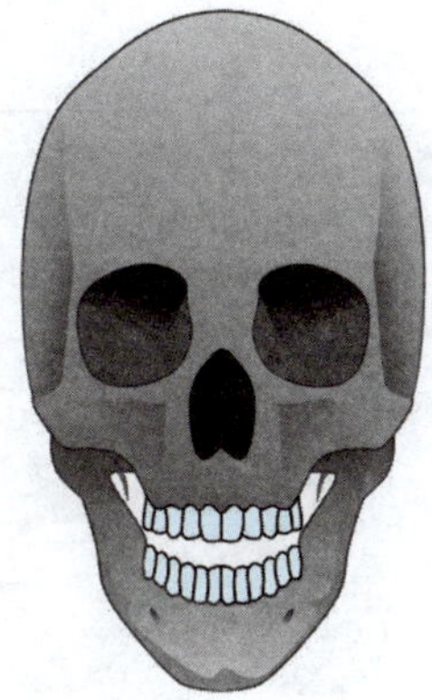

--------------------- ---------------------

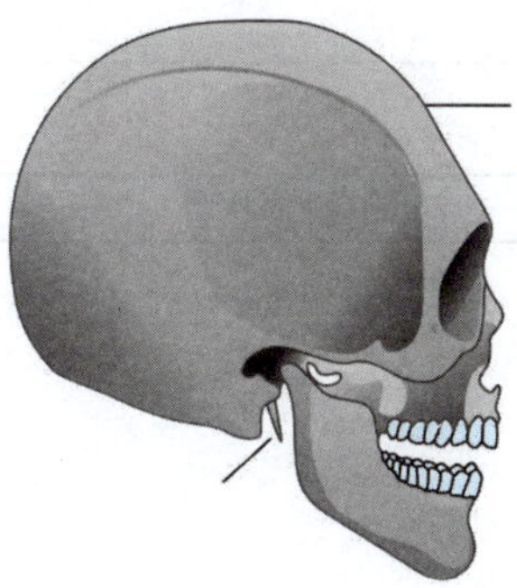

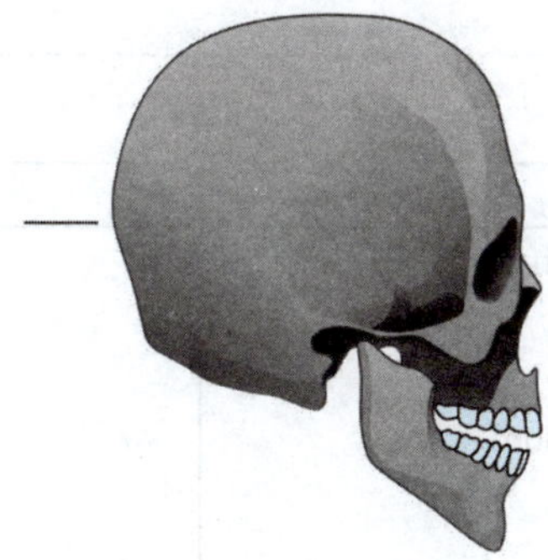

--------------------- ---------------------

Sl. No.	Trait	Male	Female
1.	Forehead		
2.	Orbit		
3.	Supraorbital ridge		
4.	Zygomatic arch		
5.	Frontonasal angle		
6.	Mastoid process		
7.	Digastric groove		
8.	Parietal eminence		
9.	Chin		
10.	Palate		

EXAMINATION OF BONES (SEX)

Pelvis:

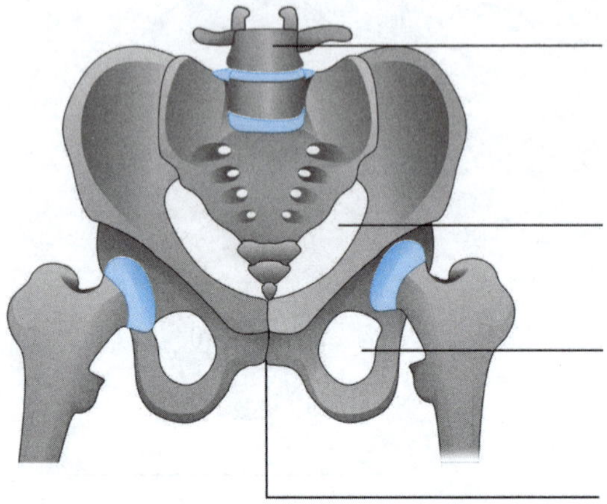

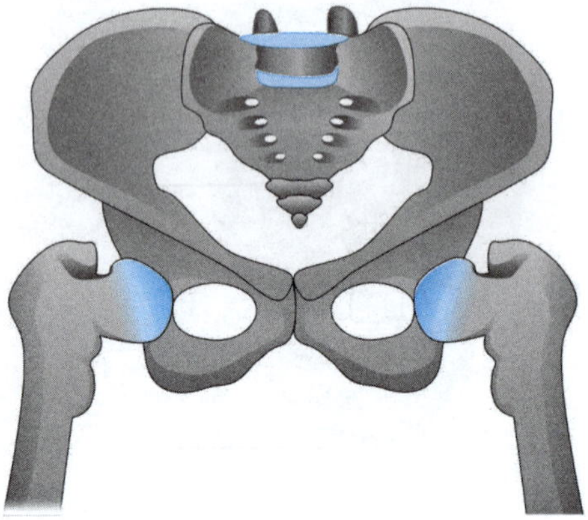

Sl. No.	Trait	Male	Female
1.	Shape		
2.	Ilium		
3.	Pre-auricular sulcus		
4.	Acetabulum		
5.	Obturator foramen		
6.	Greater sciatic notch		
7.	Subpubic angle		
8.	Pelvic brim		

DETERMINATION FROM BONES (SEX)

Male Hip Bone (Draw):

Female Hip Bone (Draw):

HIP BONE **Date..............**

Sl. No.	*Trait*	*Male*	*Female*

DETERMINATION FROM BONES (SEX)

Male Mandible (Draw):

Female Mandible (Draw):

MANDIBLE **Date..............**

Sl. No.	*Trait*	*Male*	*Female*

DETERMINATION FROM BONES (SEX)

Male Sacrum (Draw):

Female Sacrum (Draw):

SACRUM **Date...............**

Sl.No.	*Trait*	*Male*	*Female*

EXAMINATION OF BONES (AGE)

Estimation of age from closure of fontanelle of skull:

Fontanelle	*Closes at*
Anterior fontanelle	
Posterior fontanelle	
Anterolateral fontanelle	
Posterolateral fontanelle	

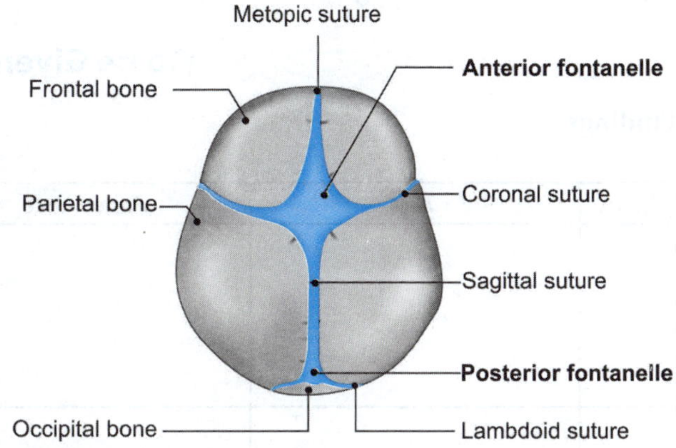

Age estimation from the given bone:

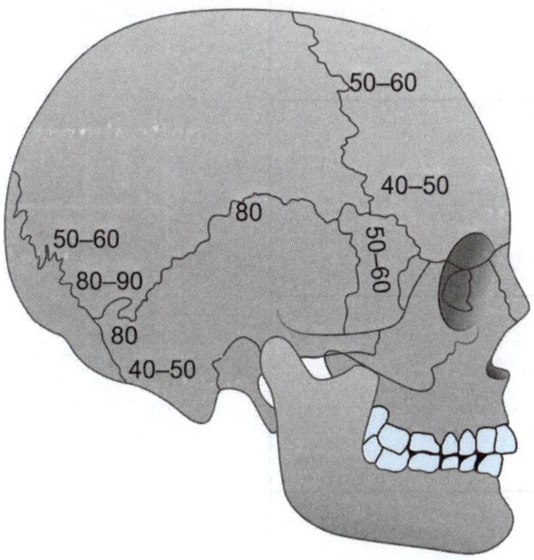

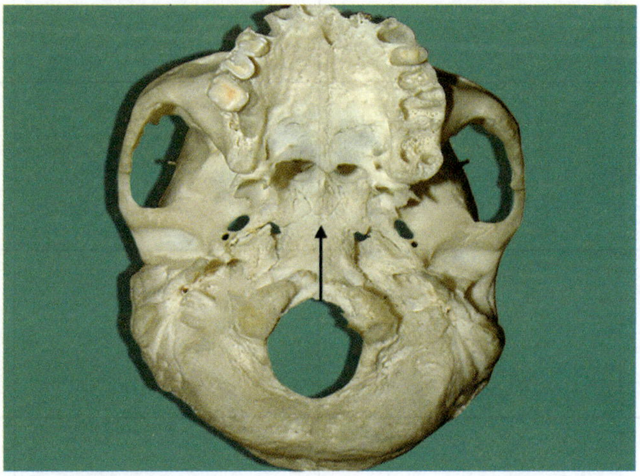

Findings

Sl. No.	*Trait*	*Appearance*	*Closure*	*Inference*

Opinion

EXAMINATION OF BONES (AGE)

Age estimation from the given bone:

(To be Given by the Teacher)

Findings

Sl. No.	Trait	Appearance	Closure	Inference

Opinion

EXAMINATION OF BONES (AGE)

Age estimation from the given bone:

(To be Given by the Teacher)

Findings

Sl. No.	*Trait*	*Appearance*	*Closure*	*Inference*

Opinion

EXAMINATION OF BONES (AGE)

Age estimation from the given bone:

(To be Given by the Teacher)

Findings

Sl. No.	*Trait*	*Appearance*	*Closure*	*Inference*

Opinion

EXAMINATION OF BONES (AGE)

Age estimation from the given bone:

(To be Given by the Teacher)

Findings

Sl. No.	Trait	Appearance	Closure	Inference

Opinion

EXAMINATION OF BONES (STATURE)

Bone	*Pan (1924) Hindus of Bengal, Bihar and Odisha*		*Mehta and Thomas, Mysuru*		*Nat (1931) UP*	*Siddiqi and Shah (1944), Punjab*	*Singh and Sohal, Punjab East*
	Males	*Females*	*Males*	*Females*	*Males*	*Males*	*Males*
Femur	3.82	3.8	3.1	3.75	3.7	3.6	3.37
Tibia	4.49	4.46	4.39	-	4.48	4.2	4.18
Fibula	4.46	4.43	4.44	4.45	4.48	4.4	4.35
Humerus	5.31	5.31	5.08	5.32	5.3	5.0	4.97
Radius	6.38	6.7	6.01	6.25	6.4	6.3	6.43
Ulna	6.0	6.0	6.4	6.85	6.3	6.0	5.93

Exercise: Estimate the stature of the individual from the supplied bones.
Use osteometric board for measuring the length of the bone after identifying its sex.

Femur

Tibia

Fibula

Humerus

Radius

Ulna

EXAMINATION OF BONES (RACE) AND DIFFERENT INDICES
Some Important Formulae for Identification of Skeletal Remains

Race

1. Cephalic Index (CI) = ———————— × 100

Skull type	*Cephalic index*	*Race*
Dolicocephalic (Long-headed)	....	....
Mesaticephalic (Medium-headed)	....	....
Brachycephalic (Short-headed)	....	....

2. Height Index (HI) = ———————— × 100

3. Nasal Index (NI) = ———————— × 100

Sex

1. Orbital Index = ———————— × 100

2. Sternal Index = ———————— × 100

3. Sacral Index = ———————— × 100

4. Ishiopubic Index = ———————— × 100

STUDY OF DENTITION

Temporary Set

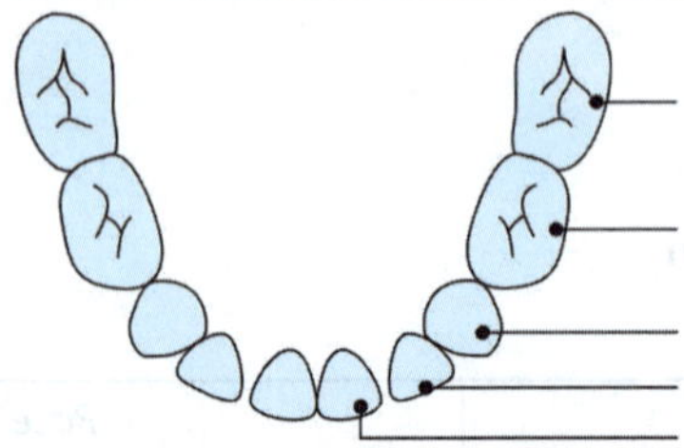

Tooth	Age of eruption

Permanent Set

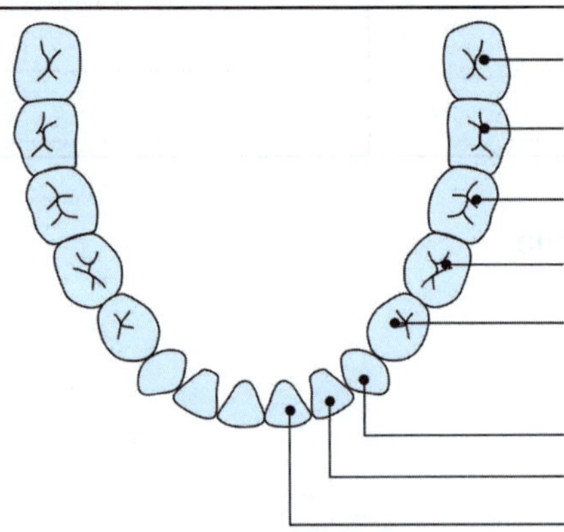

Tooth	Age of eruption

DIFFERENCES BETWEEN TEMPORARY AND PERMANENT TEETH

Trait	Temporary teeth	Permanent teeth
Size		
Direction		
Colour		
Neck		
Root		
Ridges		

STUDY OF HAIRS AND FIBRES

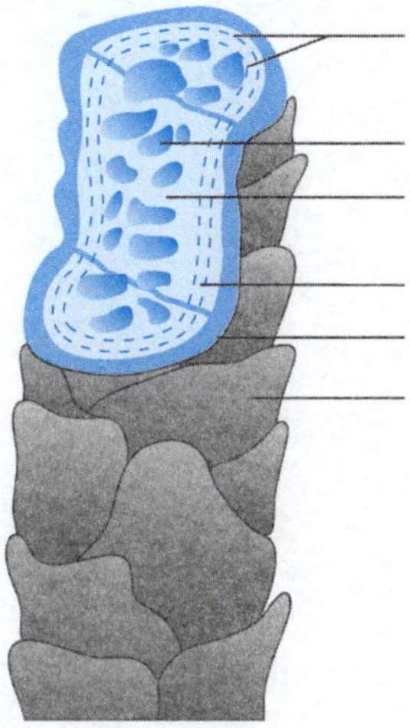

Differences between Human and Animal Hair

Features	*Human hair*	*Animal hair*
	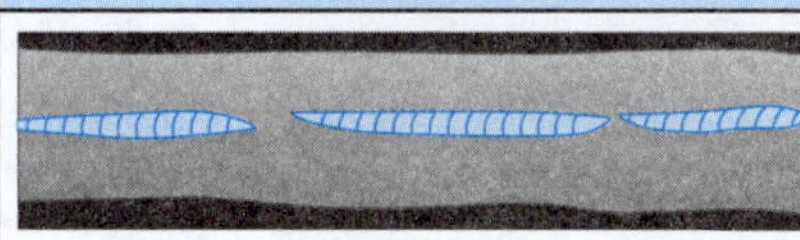	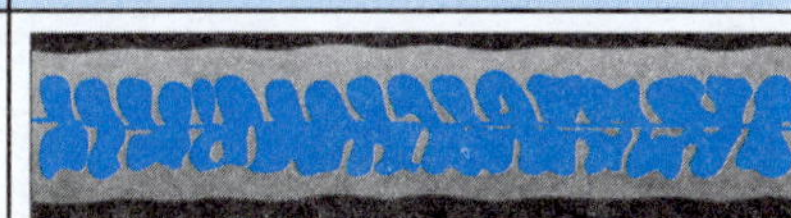
Diameter		
Cuticular scales		
Cortex		
Medulla		
Medullary index		
Pigment		
Precipitin test		

STUDY OF HAIRS AND FIBRES
Features of Hair Root, Tip and Shaft

HAIR ROOT

Naturally Fallen Hair

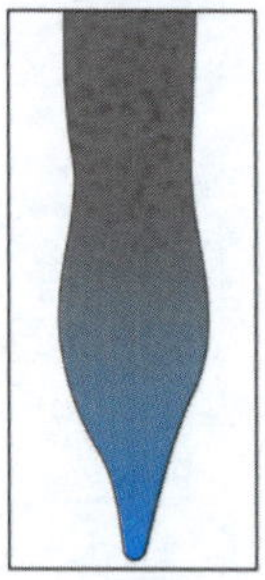

Forcibly Pulled Out

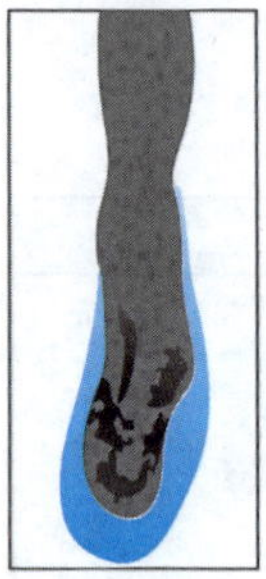

HAIR TIP

Sharp Cut

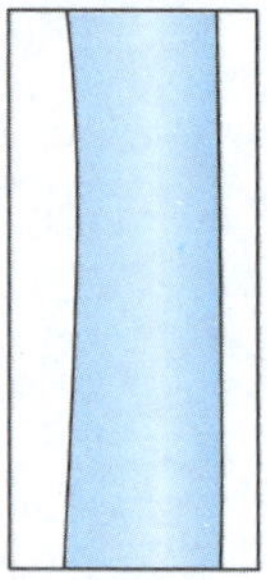

Crushed

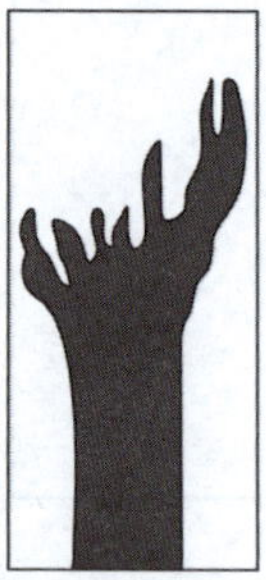

Singed

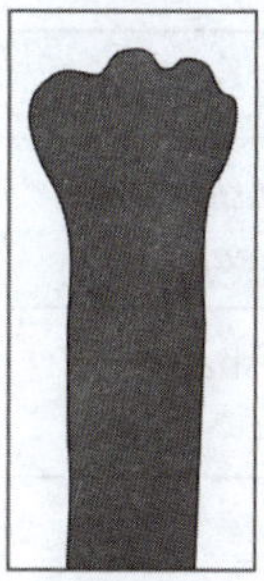

HAIR SHAFT

Dyed

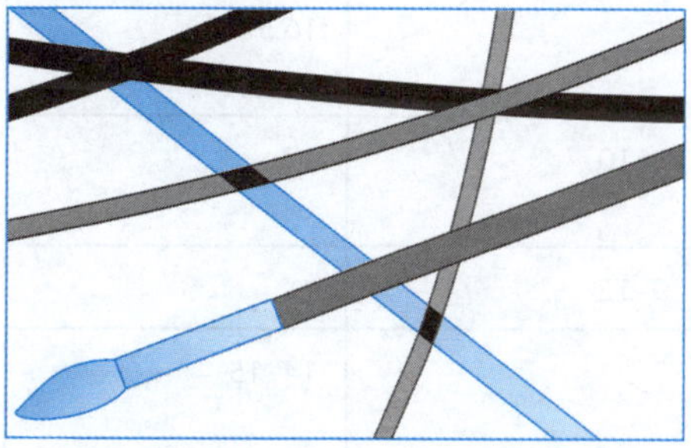

Infestations

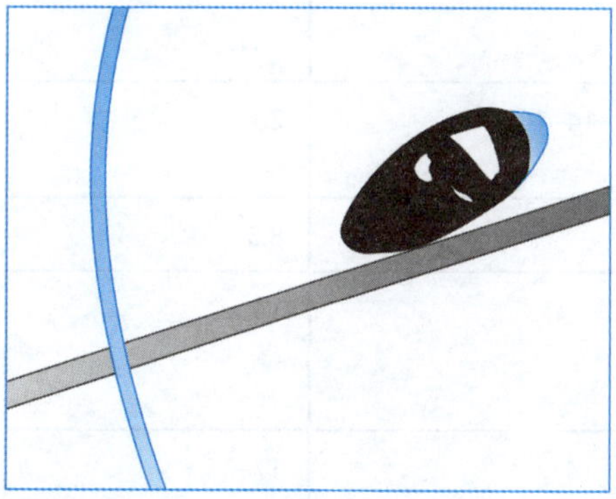

Others

GALSTAUN CHART*

X-rays	Epiphysis-cartilage of the joint	Male		Female	
		Appearance (Years)	Fusion (Years)	Appearance (Years)	Fusion (Years)
Elbow joint	• Medial epicondyle	7	16 with shaft	5	14 with shaft
	• Lateral epicondyle	12	11–16	10	10–12
	• Tip of olecranon	11–13	17	9–12	15
	• Radial head	8	16	6	14
Wrist joint	• Lower end of radius	1	16–17	1	16.5–18
	• Lower end of ulna	10–11	18	8–10	17
	• Pisiform bone	12–17	–	9–12	–
	• Head of 1st metacarpal	4	16–18	3	14–15
	• Distal ends of other metacarpals	3–4	16–18	2–3	14–15
Clavicle	• Sternal/medial end	15–19	22	14–16	20
Pelvis	• Ischiopubic rami	–	8.5	–	8.5
	• Disappearance of triradiate cartilage	–	15–16	–	14
	• Iliac crest	17	19–20	14	17–19
	• Ischial tuberosity	16–18	20	14–16	20
	• Head of femur	1	16–19	1	14–15
	• Greater trochanter	–	17	–	14
	• Lesser trochanter	–	15–17	–	15

*Ref: Mathiharan K, Patnaik AK. MODI's Medical Jurisprudence and Toxicology. 23rd Edition, LexisNexis Butterworths. 2005: 895-951.

X-RAY

Opine about age of the male subject after going through his skiagram

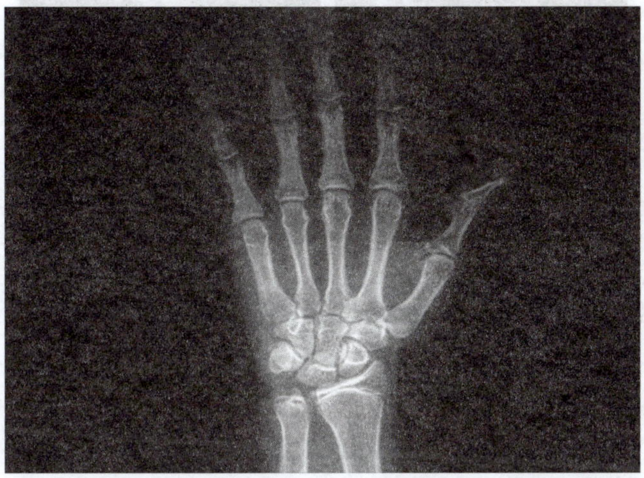

Trait	*Age of appearance*	*Observation (Appeared or not)*	*Age of fusion*	*Observation (Fused or not)*

Final opinion:

From the above observations, I am of the opinion that age of the subject is above .... years and below .... years, on the date of radiological examination.

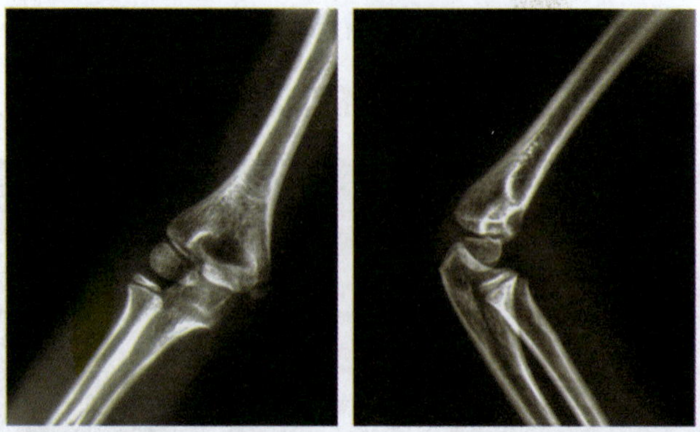

Trait	*Age of appearance*	*Observation (Appeared or not)*	*Age of fusion*	*Observation (Fused or not)*

Final opinion:

From the above observations, I am of the opinion that age of the subject is above .... years and below .... years, on the date of radiological examination.

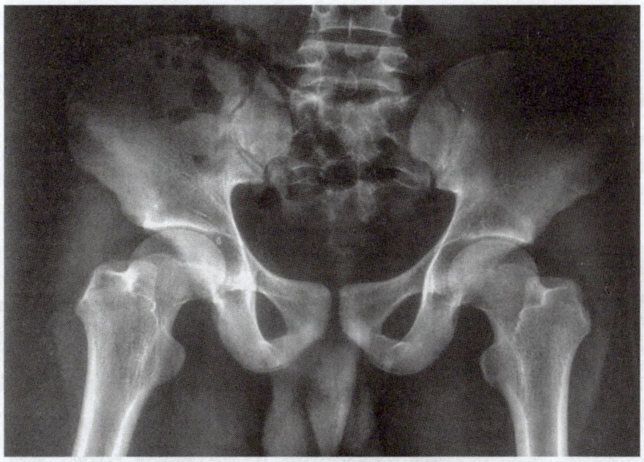

Trait	Age of appearance	Observation (Appeared or not)	Age of fusion	Observation (Fused or not)

Final opinion:

From the above observations, I am of the opinion that age of the subject is above .... years and below .... years, on the date of radiological examination.

X-RAY PROBLEMS

1. A Subinspector brought a girl to you with history of alleged sexual assault four hours back. She was recovered from an abandoned house roadside in unconscious condition. After gaining consciousness, she told to be 17 years old. You prescribed X-ray of elbow, wrist and pelvis to confirm her age. Give your opinion regarding her age from the skiagrams given below.

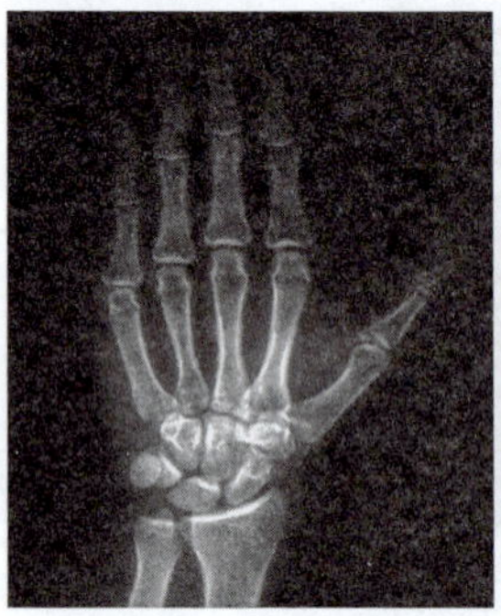
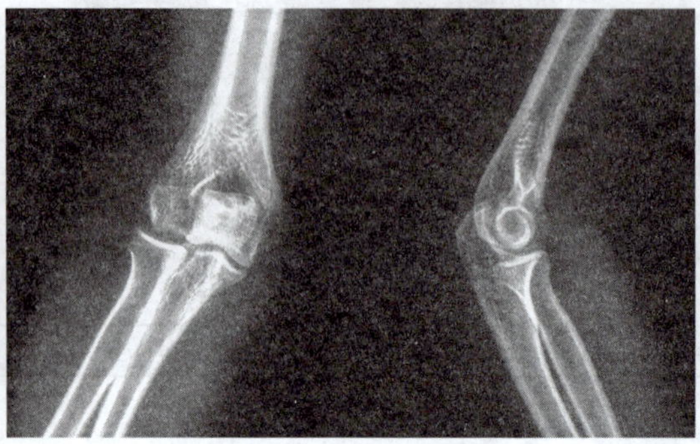
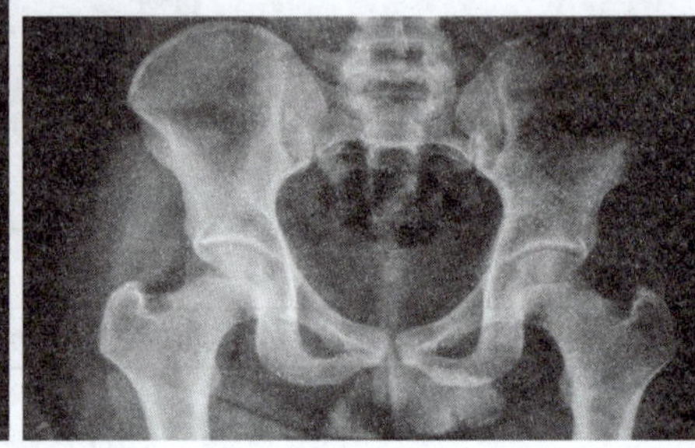

Format of Writing

Trait	*Age of appearance*	*Observation (Appeared or not)*	*Age of fusion*	*Observation (Fused or not)*

Final opinion:

From the above observations, I am of the opinion that age of the subject is above .... years and below .... years, on the date of radiological examination.

PROBLEMS ON THANATOLOGY

Exercise on Estimation of Time Since Death

1. Mr A, a 45-year-old gentleman, took his dinner at about 9 pm on 3rd June. After that, he went out for a night stroll. He usually returns home within 1 hour, but on that particular night, there was no trace of him. The worried family members informed police. After searching for considerable time, his dead body was discovered at around 7 am on 4th June, in a nearby bush. During postmortem (PM), which took place at about 2 pm on 4th June, the autopsy surgeon opined that he died due to manual strangulation. He also observed that there was presence of rigor mortis all over the body, stomach contains about 250 g partly digested food (rice and vegetables identifiable), presence of PM staining on dependent parts of body, and this does not change after change of position of body. Body was not kept in cool chamber at any time before PM. Investigating officer has made a further query to the autopsy surgeon regarding the time of death of Mr A. As an autopsy surgeon, how will you proceed to give an opinion on time since death in this case?

Sl. No.	*Observation*	*Inference*	*Reasoning*

2. Mrs B, a 65-year-old widow, lived all alone in a rented flat. She suffers from various diseases including DM and HTN. From the early part of August, her neighbours did not see her outside her flat. On 7th August, the neighbors found a foul smell coming from her flat. They informed police, and police broke the door into the flat, and found her lying dead on her bed, in a highly decomposed state. They sent the body for autopsy which started at about 2 pm on the same day. Autopsy surgeon observed that her body is in an advanced state of decomposition—her body is swollen and blacked; eyes swollen, tongue swollen, blackened and protruded; evidence of skin peeling at places with degloving of skin of right hand; hairs and nails have become loose, but have partially fallen off. All the viscera are in an advanced state of decomposition, although they can be identified individually. Brain has become liquefied into a pultaceous mass. As an autopsy surgeon, how will you proceed to give an opinion on time since death in this case?

Sl. No.	*Observation*	*Inference*	*Reasoning*

GUIDELINES FOR FILLING UP REPORT ON ESTIMATION OF AGE

- **Name of the Hospital:** ....
- **Report/Memo no.:** ....
- **Time of Examination:** ....
- **Reference:** ....
  - **In criminal cases:** ....
  - **In civil cases where the subject was sent to Department of FMT via Swastha Bhawan and MSVP Office of the concerned Medical College and Hospital:** ....
- **Recent passport size color photograph of the subject, to be attested by examining Medical Officer:** Paste passport size color photograph of the subject and attest it with your full signature and official stamp.
- **Name:** Write down the full name of the subject mentioned in concerned requisition.
- **Sex:** Male/female/third sex (in cases of transgender and transsexuals)
- **Stated age:** As stated by the subject
- **Name of the person who brought and identified the subject before Medical Officer:**
  - **In criminal cases:** ....
  - **In civil cases: Name of the person who was authorized by the concerned authority who applied to the Swastha Bhawan for estimation of age of the subject.** In such cases, authorization letter is required from the concerned authority certifying that the person will identify the subject before Medical Officer during examination. Attested (attested by concerned authority) photograph and signature of the person who will identify the subject must be present in authorization letter, e.g. Mr ABC, Assistant Engineer, PWD civil (where PWD Civil is the concerned authority who applied to the Swastha Bhawan for estimation of age of his employee)
- **Informed Consent for examination obtained from:**
  - If the subject himself or herself can give legally valid consent, then write his or her name. If the subject cannot give legally valid consent due to any reason, then take consent from parents or legal guardians.
  - Consent form must be enclosed with this report.
- **Examination done in presence of male/female attendant:**
  - If the subject is male: Write down the name of male attendant present during examination with his designation, e.g. Mr PQR, GDA, Department of Forensic Medicine and Toxicology: ....
  - If the subject is female: Write down the name of female attendant present during examination with her designation, e.g. Mrs PQR, GDA, Department of Forensic Medicine and Toxicology: ....
  - If the subject is female and no female attendant is present in Dept: you can apply for the same to the MSVP or to the Principal of the concerned Institution who can arrange a female attendant to be present during examination.
- **Identification marks:** Mention at least two identification marks of the subject, e.g.
  - One black mole of size 0.2″ × 0.1″ present over anterior aspect of left forearm, 3″ below anterior aspect of left elbow joint and 0.2″ lateral to anterior midline of that forearm.
  - One hypopigmented, glistening, nontender linear scar measuring 0.4″ × 0.1″ directed almost obliquely, present over right side of forehead, being situated 0.5″ above right supraorbital ridge and 0.6″ right to midline.
- **Height and weight:** Mention in your report accordingly.
- **BMI:** Weight in kg/height in meters^2.

- **Based on BMI note the nutritional status of the subject** because the terms well nourished, moderately nourished, poorly nourished might have subjective variations, and it is recommended not to use these terms.
  - Underweight (*BMI*< 18.5)
  - Normal (*BMI:* 18.5–22.9)
  - Overweight (*BMI:* 23–24.9)
  - Obese type 1 (*BMI:* 25–29.9)
  - Obese type 2 (*BMI:* ≥30)
  - Obese type 3 (*BMI* >50)
- **Secondary Sexual Characteristics: Refer to your report and tick the appropriate one.**
  - **Tanner staging of pubic hair in both sexes:**
    - **Tanner's stage I:** No pubic hair at all (prepubertal) **(typically age 10 and younger)**
    - **Tanner's stage II:** Small amount of long, downy hair with slight pigmentation at the base of the penis and scrotum (males) or on the labia majora (females) **(10–11.5)**
    - **Tanner's stage III:** Hair becomes more coarse and curly, and begins to extend laterally **(11.5–13)**
    - **Tanner's stage IV:** Adult-like hair quality, extending across pubis but sparing medial thighs **(13–15)**
    - **Tanner's stage V:** Hair extends to medial surface of the thighs **(15+)**
  - **Tanner staging of breast development in females:**
    - **Tanner's stage I**: No glandular tissue, areola follows the skin contours of the chest (prepubertal) (typically age 10 and younger)
    - **Tanner's stage II:** Breast bud forms, with small area of surrounding glandular tissue; areola begins to widen with increase in pigmentation (10–11.5)
    - **Tanner's stage III: [one mound stage]** Breast begins to become more elevated, and extends beyond the borders of the areola, which continues to widen but remains in contour with surrounding breast (11.5–13)
    - **Tanner's stage IV: [two mound stage]** Increased breast size and elevation; areola and papilla **form a secondary mound projecting from the contour of the surrounding breast (secondary mounding of areola above the plane of breast and papilla or nipple above areola) (13–15).**
    - **Tanner's stage V: [one mound stage]** Breast reaches final adult size; areola returns to contour of the surrounding breast, with a projecting central papilla (15+)
  - **Tanner staging of male genitalia:**
    - **Tanner I:** Testicular volume less than 1.5 ml; small penis of 3 cm or less (prepubertal) (typically age nine and younger)
    - **Tanner II:** Testicular volume between 1.6 and 6 ml; skin on scrotum thins, reddens and enlarges; penis length unchanged (9–11)
    - **Tanner III:** Testicular volume between 6 and 12 ml; scrotum enlarges further; penis begins to lengthen to about 6 cm (11–12.5)
    - **Tanner IV:** Testicular volume between 12 and 20 ml; scrotum enlarges further and darkens; penis increases in length to 10 cm (12.5–14)
    - **Tanner V:** Testicular volume greater than 20 ml; adult scrotum and penis of 15 cm in length (14+)
  - **In cases of female note down the menarche (first menstrual bleeding in female):** Started how many days or years back
  - **Menopause:** In elderly female subject ask, if she had menopause (absence of menstrual periods for 12 consecutive months)

- **Wrinkling on skin**: Note whether appropriate with stated age
- **Arcus senilis:** It is a white or grey-colored opaque ring in the corneal margin (peripheral corneal opacity). It is quite commonly present in the elderly. It can also appear earlier in life as a result of hypercholesterolemia. Note whether it is present or not. If present, then mention whether it is complete or incomplete.
- **Dental examination:**
  - We have followed Palmer's notation of dental charting system where no 1 to 8 indicates permanent teeth and A to E indicates temporary teeth.
  - Count the total number of teeth present, try to differentiate between temporary and permanent ones, if the subject is in the period of mixed dentition and tick the appropriate tooth in the chart.
  - Note down the total number of teeth, number of temporary and permanent teeth.
  - Note if spacing for third molar is present after eruption of permanent 2nd molar tooth
  - Note whether any tooth is missing or broken after its eruption.
  - *Note the degree of attrition (A) and Periodontosis:*
    A0: No attrition, A1: Attrition within enamel, A2: Attrition reaching dentin
    A3: Attrition reaching dental pulp.
    P0: No Periodontosis, P1: Periodontosis just started, less than 1/3rd root is exposed, P2: 1/3rd to 2/3rd of root is exposed, P3: More than 2/3rd root is exposed.
  - **Reference chart for eruption of temporary teeth:**

Name of deciduous teeth	*Age of eruption*
Central incisor—lower	6th month
Central incisor—upper	7th month/8th month
Lateral incisor—upper	8th month/10th month
Lateral incisor—lower	9th month/12th month
1st molar	12th–14th month
Canine	18th month
2nd molar	24–30th month

  - **Reference chart for eruption of permanent teeth:**

Name of permanent teeth	*Age of eruption*
1st molar	6–7 years
Central incisors (both upper and lower)	7–8 years
Lateral incisors (both upper and lower)	8–9 years
1st premolar	9–10 years
2nd premolar	10–11 years
Canine	11–12 years
2nd molar	12–14 years
3rd molar	17–25 years or even later

  - If you have any confusion regarding whether a tooth is temporary or permanent one you can suggest for orthopantomograph (OPG) and note down your findings accordingly.

- **Radiological examination:**
  - Suggest radiological examination depending on the stated age of the subject, make a requisition for the same and hand over the requisition to the person who brought and identified the subject and take his signature.
  - In the State of West Bengal, we follow the Galstaun chart for Bengalis.
  - ***For Reference:*** Galstaun's chart (Page no. 22)
- **Opinion:** While making your opinion, you have to give due consideration on the findings of physical, dental and radiological examination because each of them depends on several criteria.
  - The estimated age may corroborate with the stated age of the subject or may not corroborate.
  - We have to keep it in mind that observations made upon the data of Galstaun chart has a range of error ± 3 years and radiological bony union is considered 2–3 years earlier than actual anatomical bony union.
  - For example, if your estimated age is above 16 years but less than 18 years and stated age of the subject is 17 years, then your estimated age corroborates with stated age of the subject, but if the subject stated his age is 19 years, then it is not corroborating with your estimated age. In such a case with inclusion of margin of error on either side, the subject's stated age can be taken into consideration.

AGE ESTIMATION REPORT

1. A bank has applied before Swastha Bhawan for fixation of the age of his employee Ratan Ghosh whose stated age is 56 years, though according to the bank he has crossed 60 years of age. Ratan has no valid documentation certifying his age. Swasthya Bhawan referred the case to MSVP of a Govt Medical College and Hospital vide Memo No: XYZ, who in turn referred the case to Department of FMT of that Hospital vide Memo No. ABC. Ratan was brought to the department by Mr Sumanta Saha, who was authorized by the Manager of the concerned bank to identify Ratan before Medical Officer. Ratan has following identification marks:
   i. One black mole present over left cheek
   ii. One whitish glistening scar on anterior aspect of left forearm.

   Physical examination revealed that he has arcus senilis completely encircling the corneal margin, greying of pubic hairs.

   Skiagram revealed complete fusion of sagittal and coronal sutures, though parietomastoid suture fusion started but not completed and xiphoid process and manubrium have fused with body of sternum.

   Based on the above-noted findings, prepare an age estimation report.

Format

Name of the Hospital: ....

Department: Forensic Medicine and Toxicology

Report on Estimation of Age

Report/Memo no.: .... **Date:** ....

Date of Examination: .... **Time of Examination:** ....

Reference: ....

Recent passport size color photograph of the subject, to be attested by examining Medical Officer

Preliminaries

1. **Name:** ....
2. **Sex:** .... (male/female/others) 3. **Stated age:** ....
4. **Name of the person who brought and identified the subject before Medical Officer:**
   Name: ....
   Designation: ....
   Signature with date: ....
5. **Informed consent for examination obtained from (Informed Consent form is enclosed with the Report):**
   Name: ....
   Signature with date: ....
6. **Examination done in presence of male/female attendant:**

Name: ....

Designation: ....

Signature with date: ....

7. Identification marks (at least two)

I...

....

II...

....

III...

....

Physical Examination

8. Height: .... **9. Weight:** .... **10. BMI:** .... (Weight in Kg/Height in meters^2)

11. Nutritional status based on BMI: (WHO criteria) [Tick the appropriate one]

A. Underweight (BMI<18.5), B. Normal (BMI: 18.5–22.9), C. Overweight (BMI: 23–24.9), D. Obese type 1 (BMI: 25–29.9), E. Obese type 2 (BMI: ≥30), F. Obese type 3 (BMI >50)

12. Secondary sexual characteristics (Tick the appropriate one)

Male	*Female*
Beard: Not appeared/soft growth/sparse/coarse/shaved in recent past *Graying*: Present/absent	Breast development: Tanner stage
Moustache: Not appeared/soft growth/sparse/coarse/shaved in recent past *Graying*: Present/absent	Axillary hair: Not appeared/soft growth/sparse/coarse/shaved in recent past Graying: Present/absent
Axillary hair: Not appeared/soft growth/sparse/coarse/shaved in recent past *Graying*: Present/absent	Pubic hair: Tanner stage Graying of pubic hair: Present/absent
Pubic hair: Tanner stage *Graying of pubic hair:* Present/absent	Menarche: Yes/no If yes how many days or years back
Penis and scrotum: Tanner stage	Menopause: Yes/no If yes how many days or years back

13. Other features:

i. *Wrinkling on skin:* Whether appropriate with stated age.......................................

ii. *Arcus senilis:* Present/absent. If present note whether it is incomplete or complete..................................

Dental Examination

Teeth:

RIGHT LEFT

14. Total number of teeth: ....

15. Total number of temporary teeth: ....

16. Total number of permanent teeth: ....

17. Spacing for third molar: ....

18. Erupted but missing tooth/broken tooth any: ....

19. Degree of attrition: ....(A0–A3)

20. Degree of periodontosis: ....(P0–P3)

21. Orthopantomograph, if required: (yes/no) If required, findings of orthopantomogram:

Radiological Examination

22. Digital X-ray examination advised: (tick the appropriate one) Ossification centres around

- i. Elbow joint (AP and lateral view)
- ii. Wrist joint (AP view)
- iii. Pelvis (AP view)
- iv. Shoulder joint (AP and lateral view)
- v. Chest (AP and lateral view showing medial end of clavicles and sternum)
- vi. Skull (AP/Towne's view and lateral view showing cranial sutures)

23. In older age group for precise calculation of fusion of ossification centres and cranial sutures [Tick, if required]:

- i. 3D-CT scan of skull showing cranial sutures
- ii. 3D-CT scan of sternum showing ossification centres

24. Requisition for radiological examination is handed over to:

Name: ....

Signature with date: ....

25. Findings on radiological examination:

- Date of radiological examination: ....
- Date of receipt of radiological plates: ....
- Place or centre of radiological examination: ....
- Plate no.: ....
- Whether identification marks mentioned in requisition for radiological examination were tallied or not: .... (Yes/No)

Sl. No.	*Part examined*	*Observations*	*Inference*

Opinion

Considering the findings of physical, dental and radiological examinations, I am of the opinion that the age of the subject identified as ....is above........................... years and below .... Years of age on the date of radiological examination, i.e. on ....with inclusion of margin of error on either side.*

....

(Full Signature of the Medical Officer with Registration No, Date and Official Seal)

*[Note: observations made upon the data of Galstaun chart has a range of error ± 3 years and radiological bony union is considered 2 to 3 years earlier than actual anatomical bony union]

MORE EXERCISE

1. Kamal, accused under Sec 376 IPC, was brought to the Department of FMT by SI Ranjit Mukherjee of Entally PS for medicolegal examination and age estimation vide Entally PS Case No 235 dated 14/10/17 under 376 IPC. Kamal was claiming he was juvenile, though according to the Police, he was 21 years of age.
   Kamal had the following particulars:
   Height: 5 feet 1 inches, weight: 51 kg.
   Identification marks:
   i. One white nontender scar over anterior aspect of right side of chest wall.
   ii. One mole over right side of forehead.
   Dental examination revealed 2nd molar teeth erupted in each quadrant, spacing were present in each quadrant Physical examination revealed pubic hairs extended to medial aspect of thigh.
   Radiological examination revealed all the ossification centres around elbow joint and wrist had fused. Ischial tuberosity had appeared and fused. Medial end of both clavicles though appeared but not fused.
   Based on the above-noted findings, prepare an age estimation report.
2. ***To be given by the teacher***

PHOTOGRAPH

In practical field of forensic medicine, frequently, photographs are in need to be interpreted in relation to medicolegal cases. Here are some exercises:

1. Describe the identifying feature visible in this photograph. What can be the possible chemical substance used while inscribing? What may be the possible causes of fading of the feature?

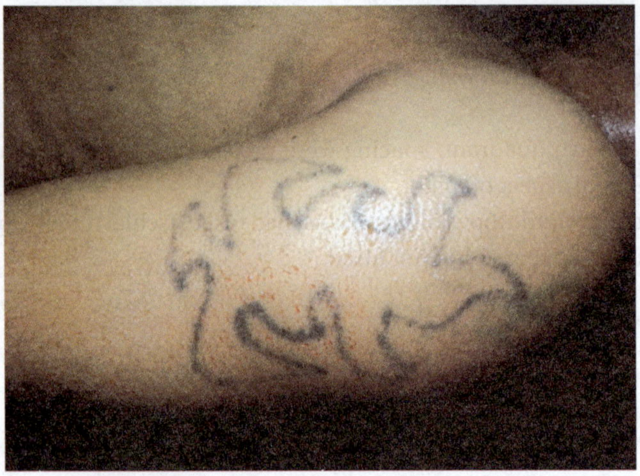

2. Identify and describe the injury visible in this photograph. From naked eye examination, ascertain the approximate time since infliction of the injury with reasoning.

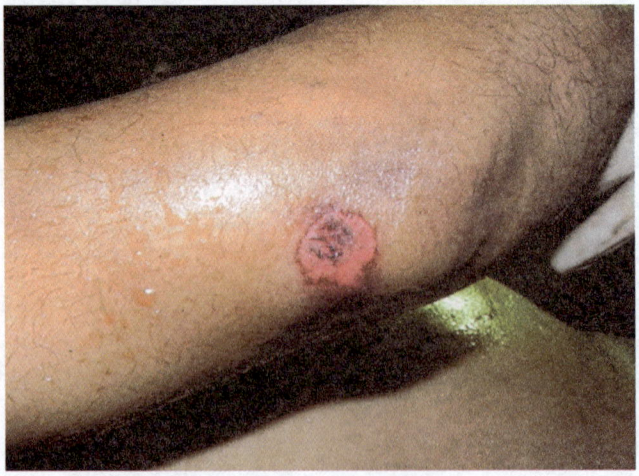

3. Identify and describe the injury visible in this photograph. From naked eye examination, ascertain the approximate time since infliction of the injury with reasoning.

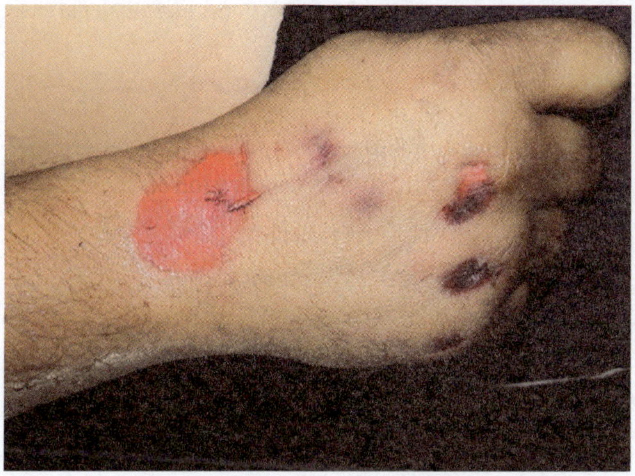

4. Identify and describe the injury visible in this photograph. From naked eye examination, ascertain the approximate time since infliction of the injury with reasoning. What may be the possible circumstances? What may be the underlying injuries that can be found in this case?

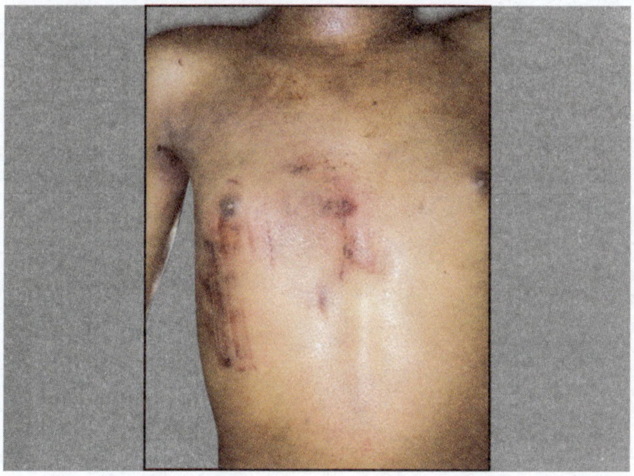

5. Identify and describe the injury visible in this photograph. Is there any evidence of medical attention present? If yes, identify that.

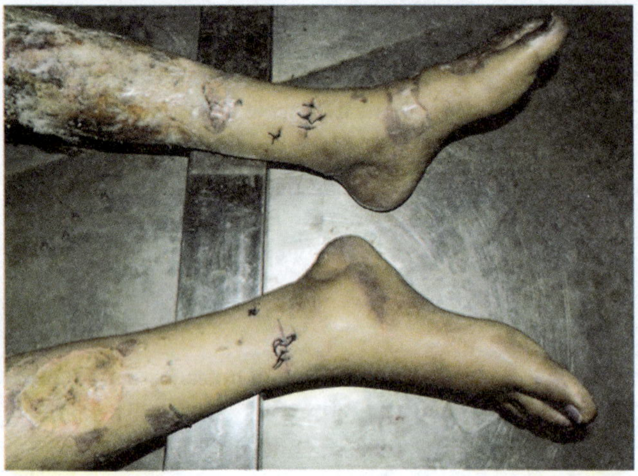

6. Identify and describe the injury visible in this photograph. From naked eye examination, ascertain the approximate time since infliction of the injury with reasoning. Why the veins are prominently visible?

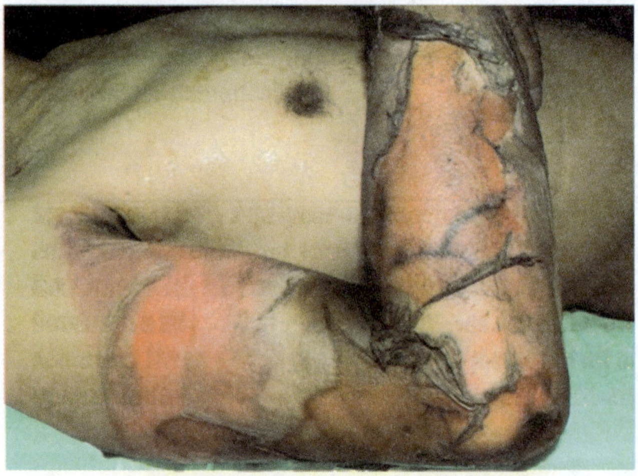

7. Identify and describe the changes occurred due to pregnancy in this photograph.

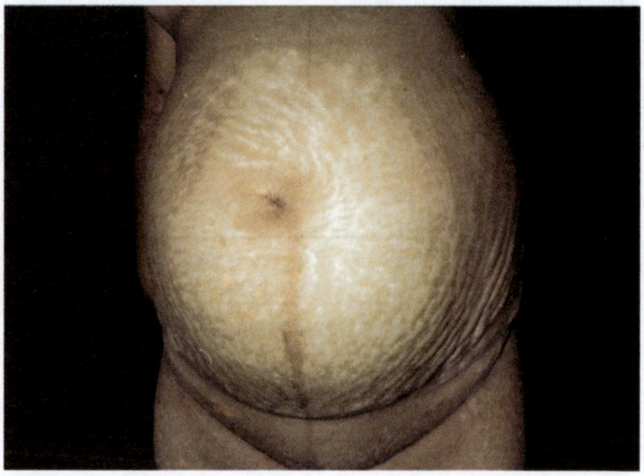

8. Identify the feature visible around the neck of the person in this picture. Describe the feature in which circumstance it can be found? What may be the possible finding after dissection?

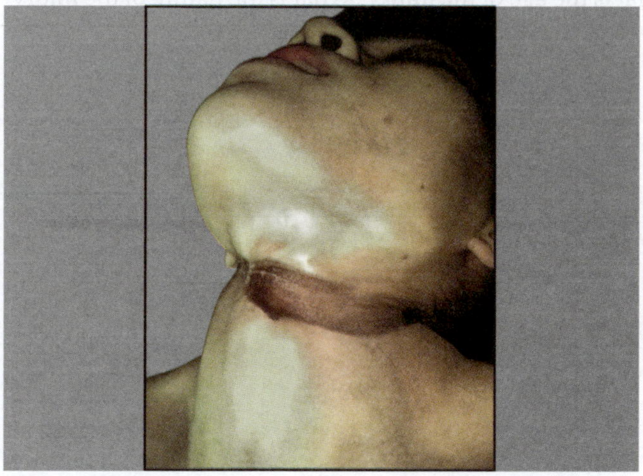

MECHANICAL INJURIES AND WEAPONS

1. Describe and identify the injury. How it is produced? What is the age of the injury? What is the nature of the injury? What is the direction of application of force?

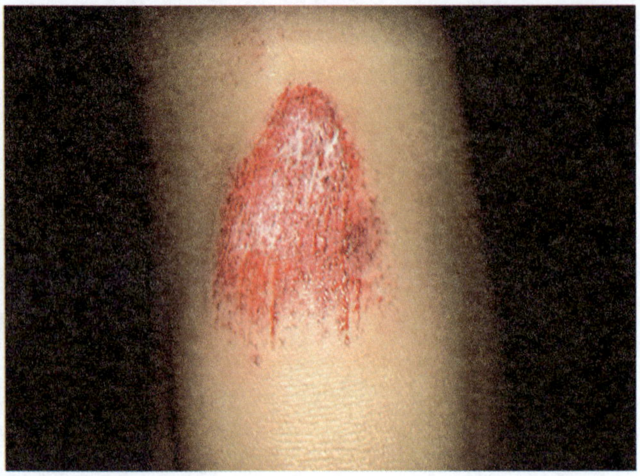

2. Describe and identify the injury. How it is produced? What is the age of the injury? What is the nature of the injury?

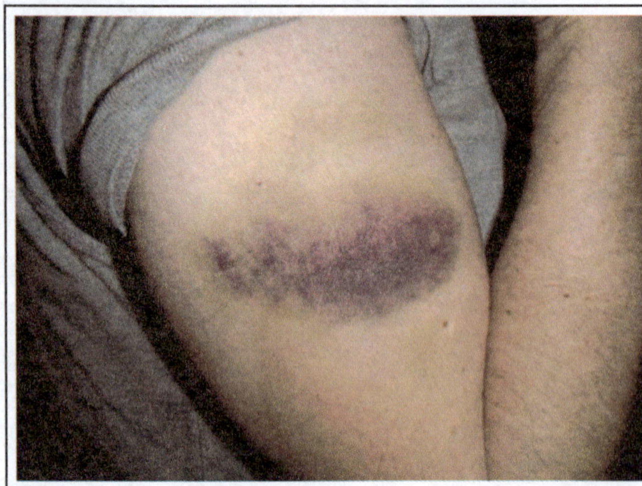

3. Describe and identify the injury. How it is produced? What is the age of the injury? What is the nature of the injury? Can you ascertain direction of application of force?

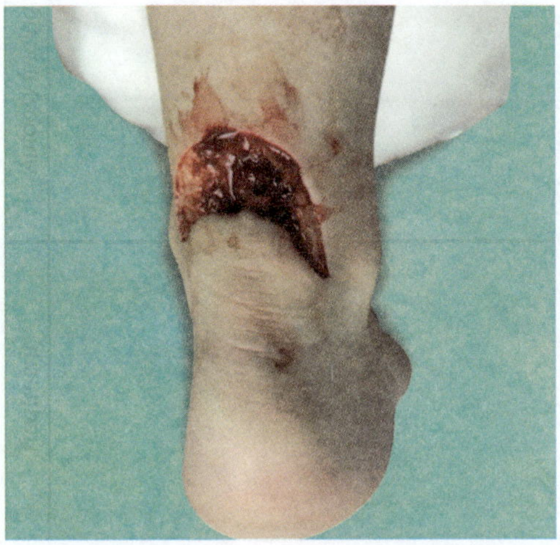

4. Identify the following types of skull fractures and write their mechanism of production and its complication. What is the nature of injury?

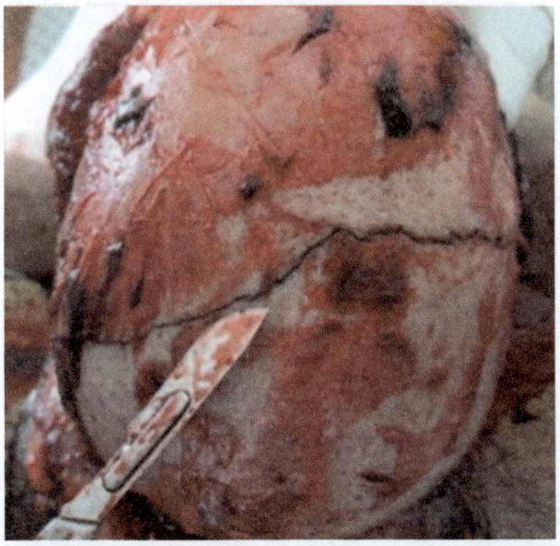

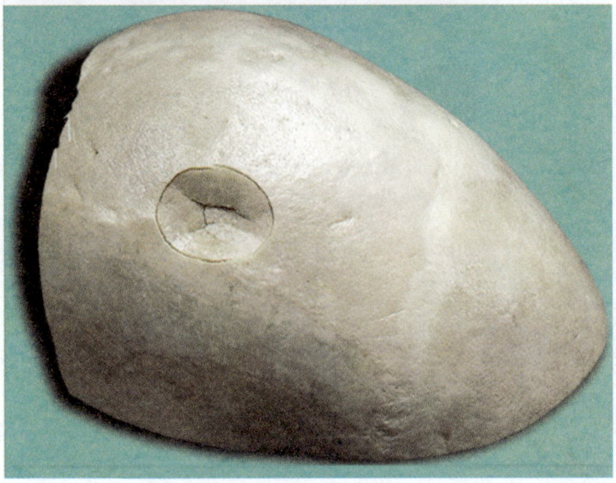

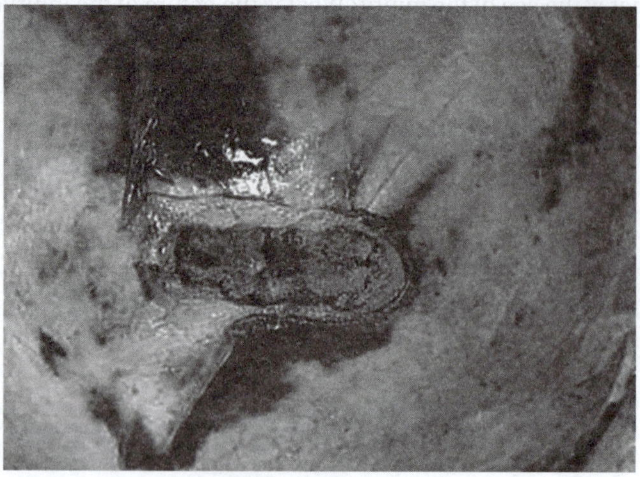

5. Identify the following signs associated with skull fractures and mention their medicolegal importance.

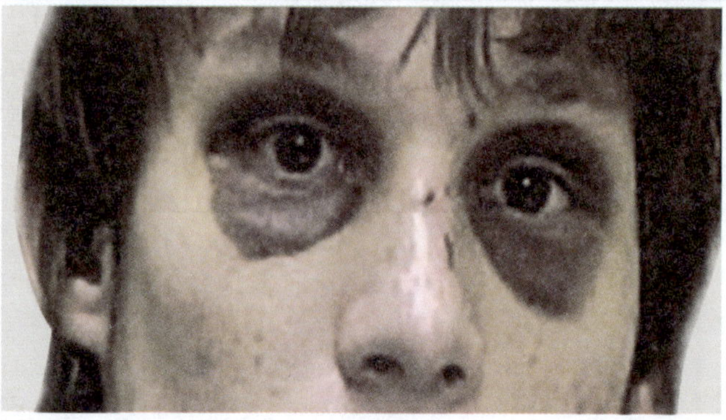

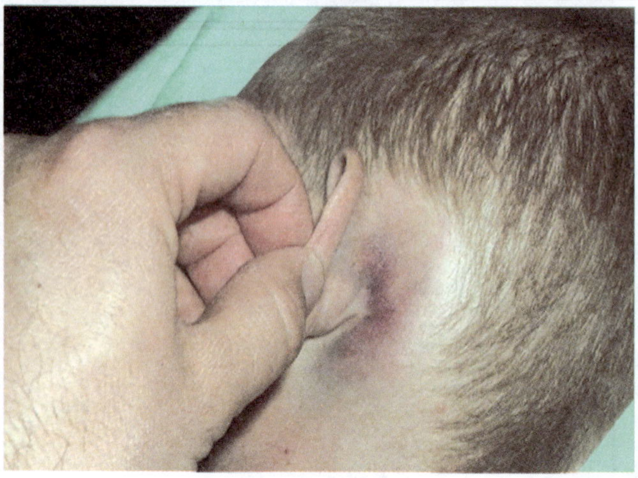

6. Describe and identify the following injuries. Write their medicolegal importance.

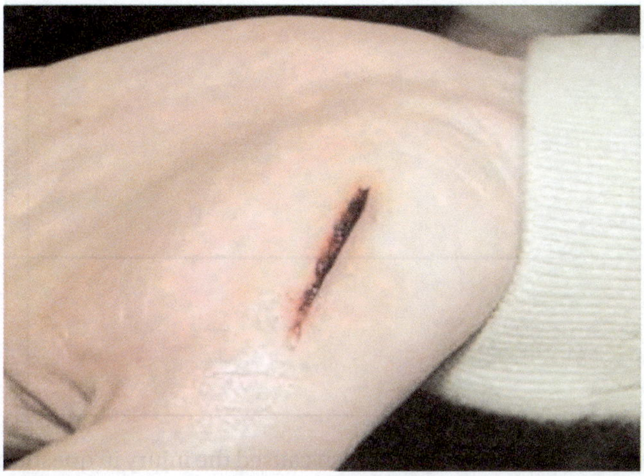

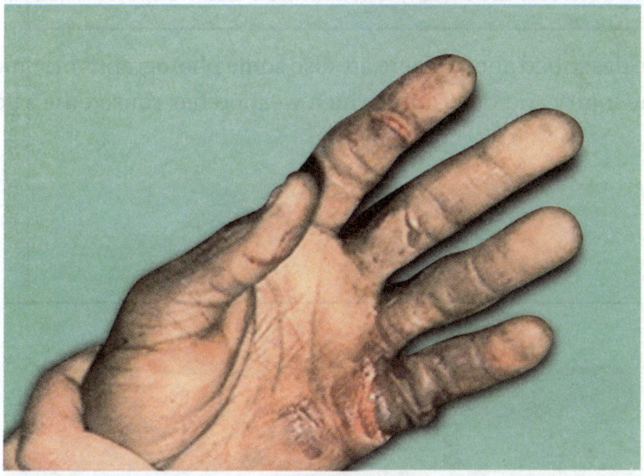

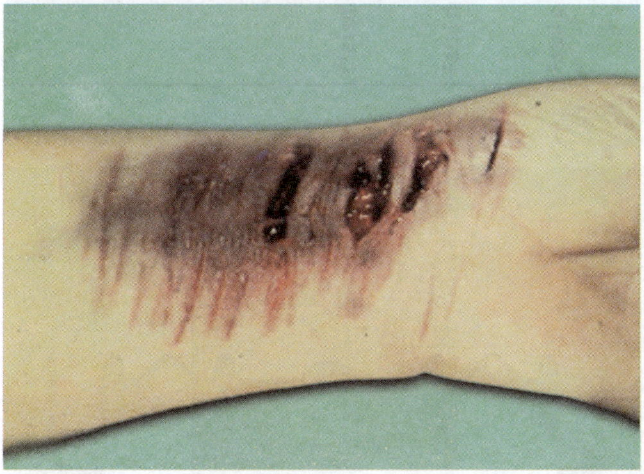

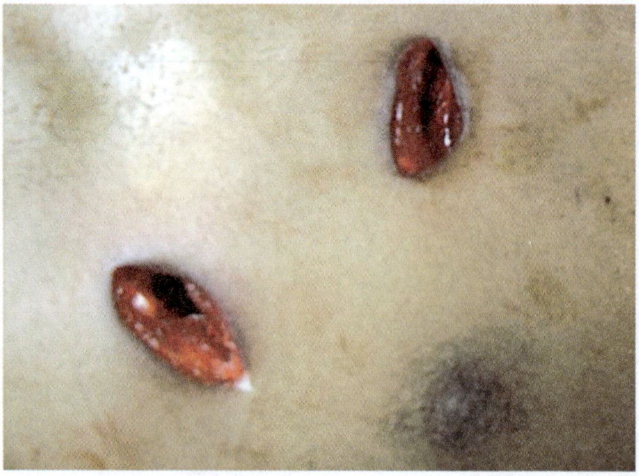

7. In practice a doctor is often asked by police or court of law to identify the weapon which caused the injury in question. So a doctor as an expert witness, must be able to correlate between the injury, he examined and weapon police has produced.

   Given below are some photographs of injuries as you have described above. There are also some photographs of some common weapons. You need to describe and identify the injury and determine which weapon has caused the said injury.

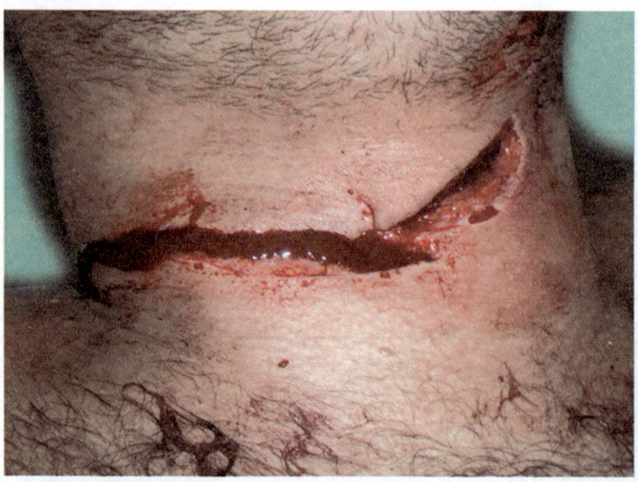

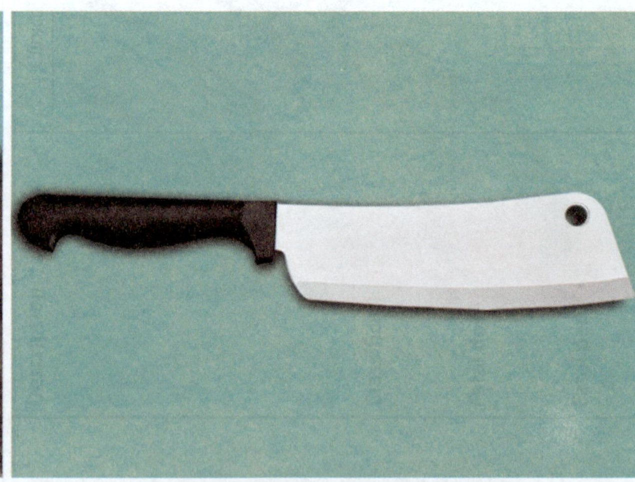

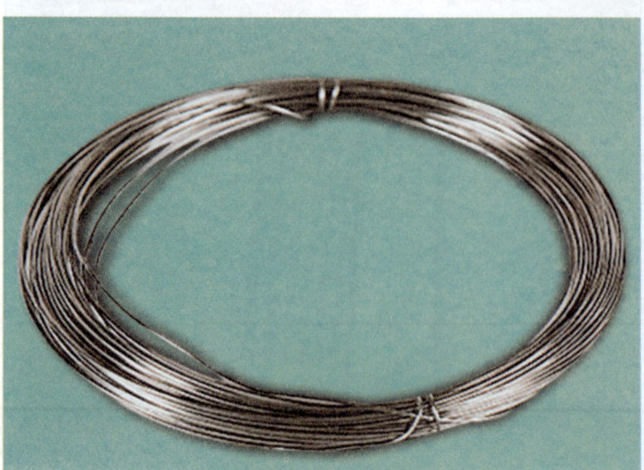

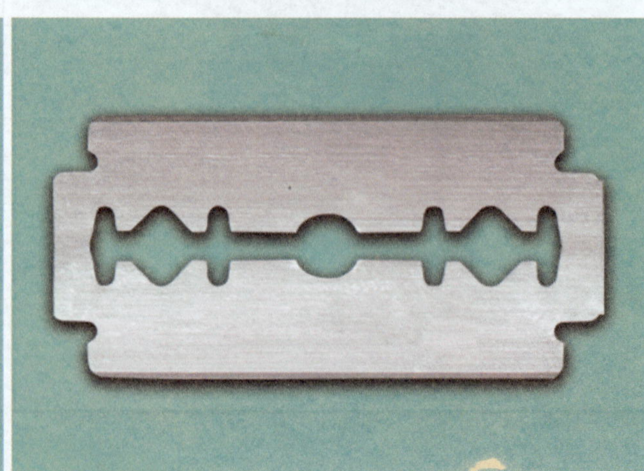

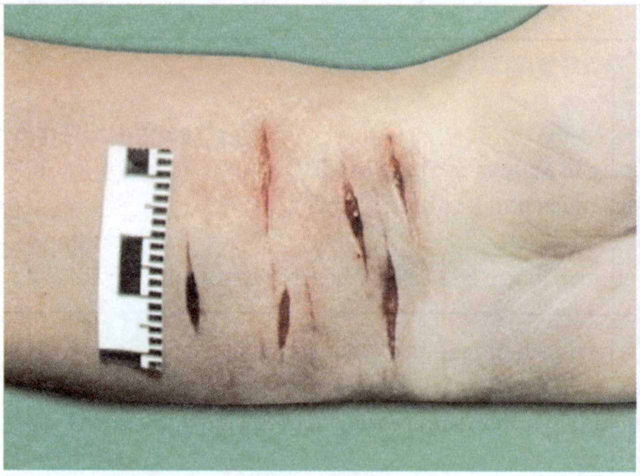

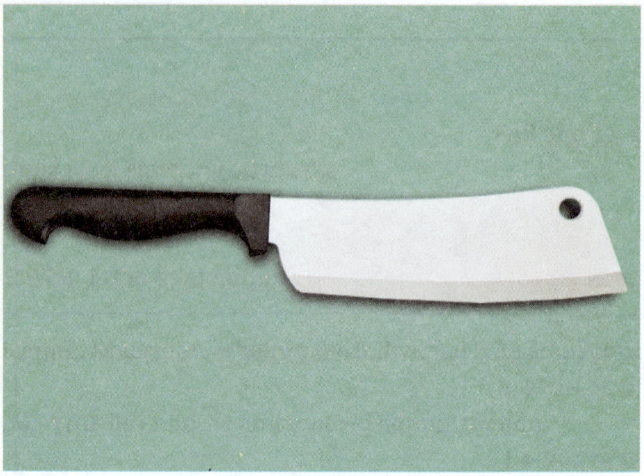

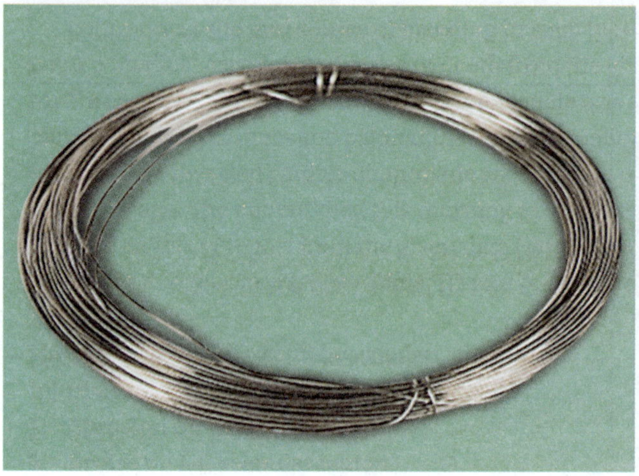

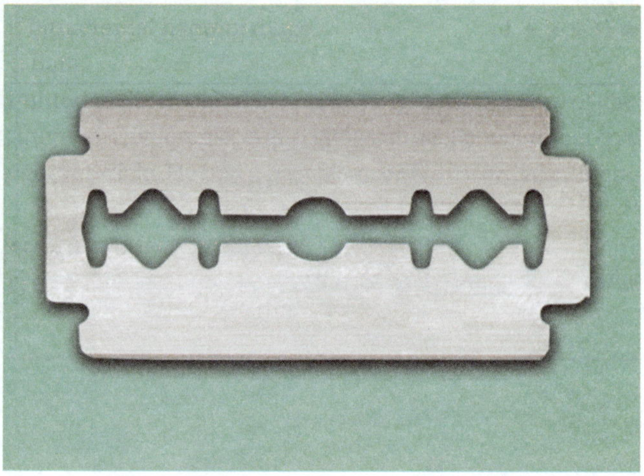

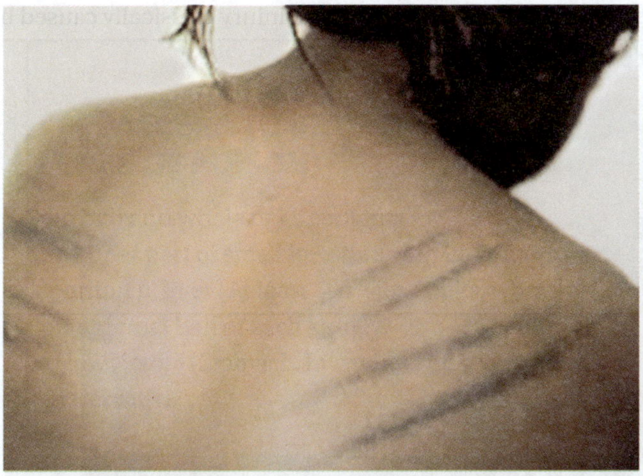

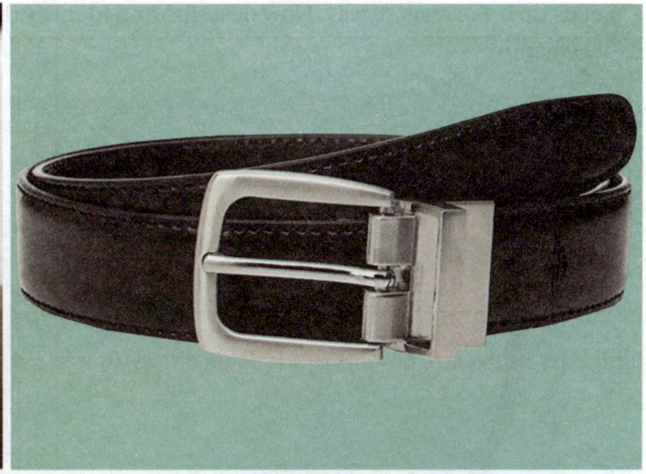

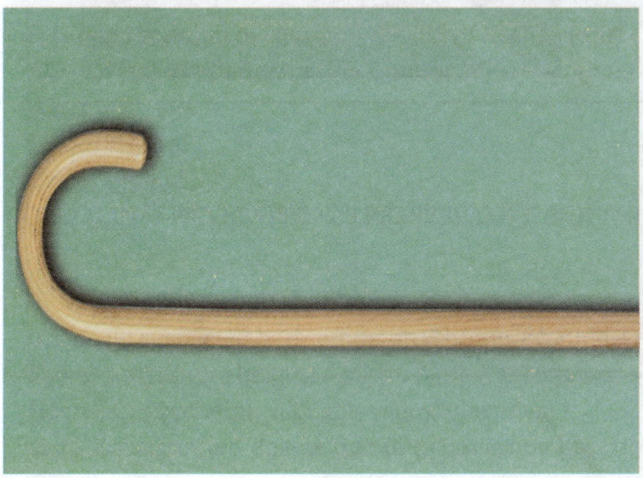

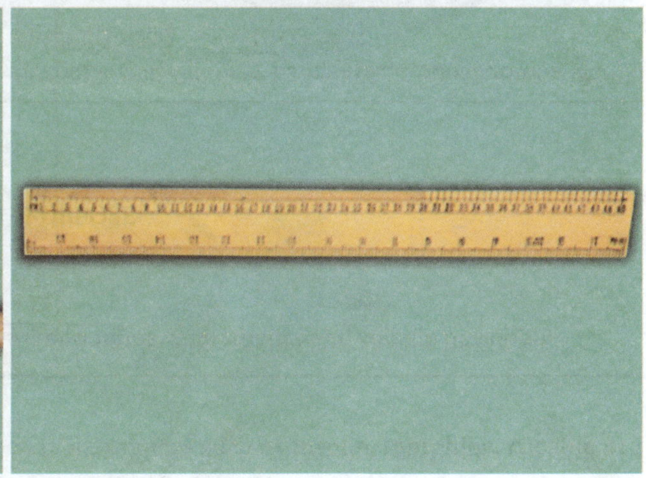

8. Let us do it the reverse way. Now describe and identify the weapon and then identify the injury classically caused by the weapon.

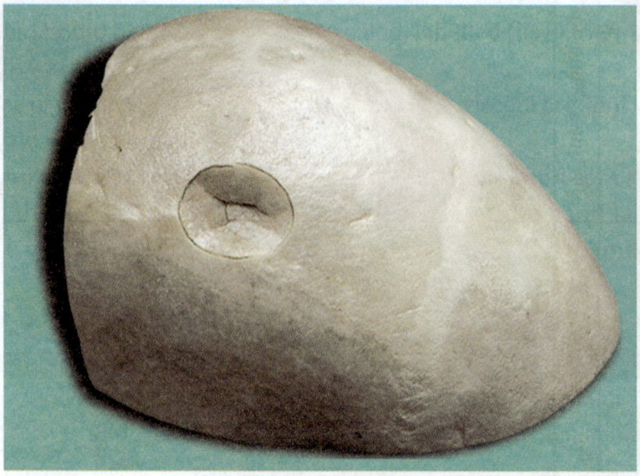

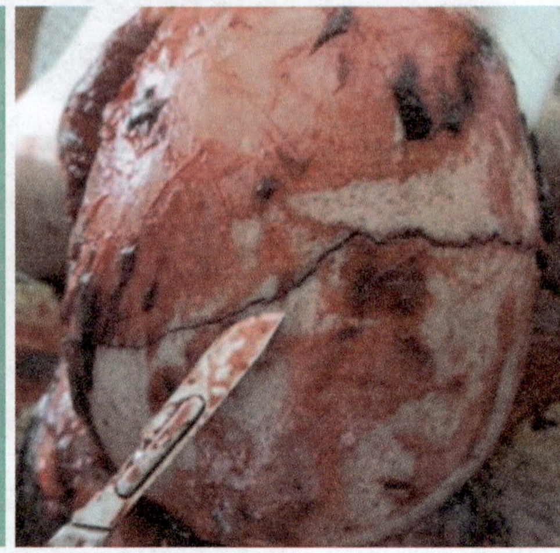

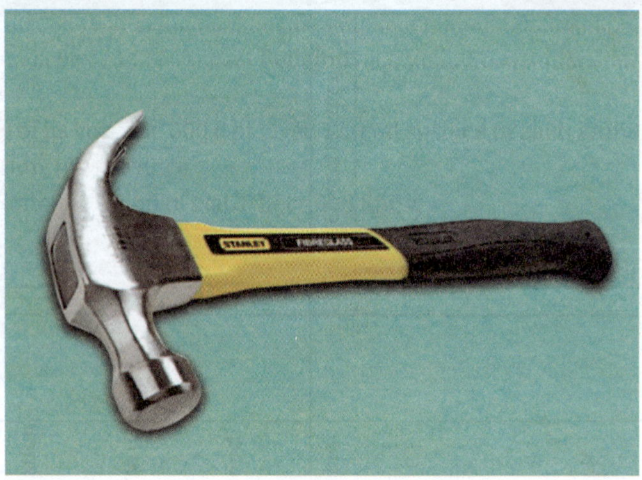

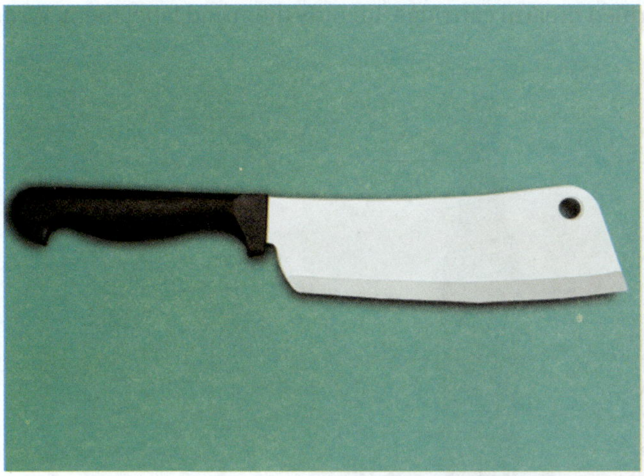

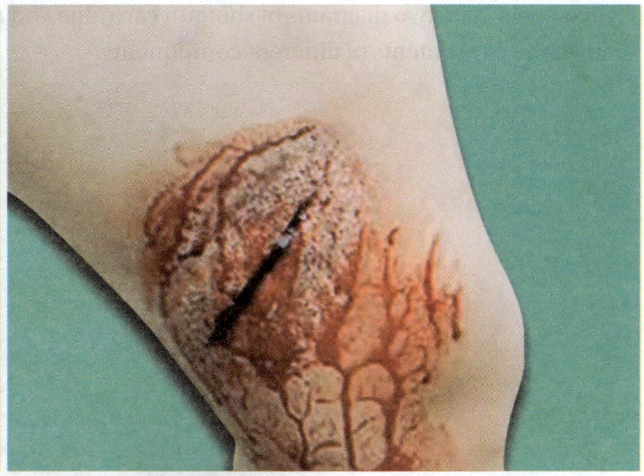

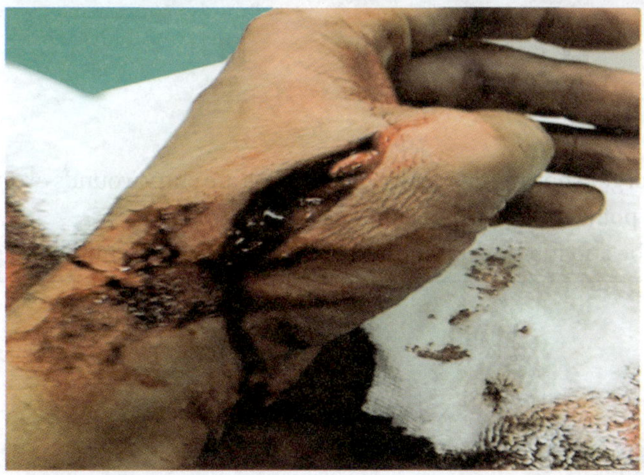

9. Given below are two diagrams of shotgun cartridge and rifled firearm cartridge. Identify them and label them. Write down the constituents of different components.

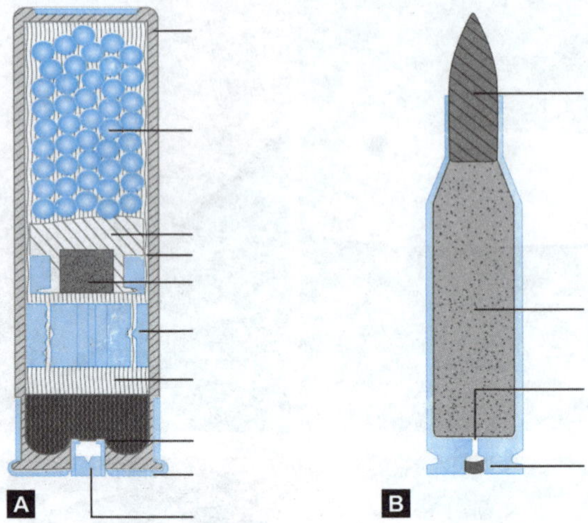

10. Few coloured photographs of gunshot injuries are given below. All are entry wounds *except one*. Identify that photograph of exit wound and give two points in support of your answer.
For the rest of them, describe and identify their different features and determine range of the shot.

Description

Inference:

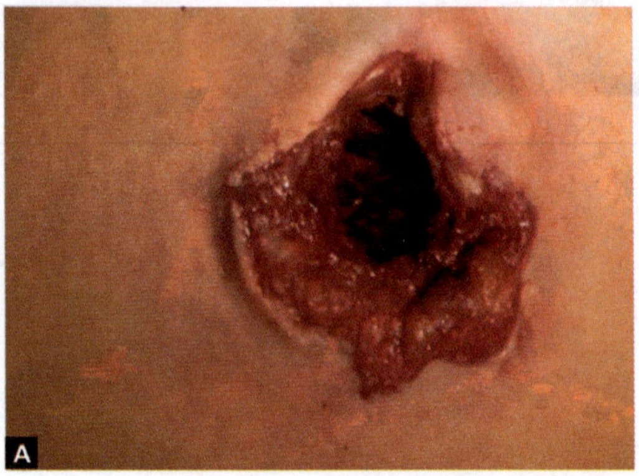

Two supporting points:

i.

ii.

Description

Inference:

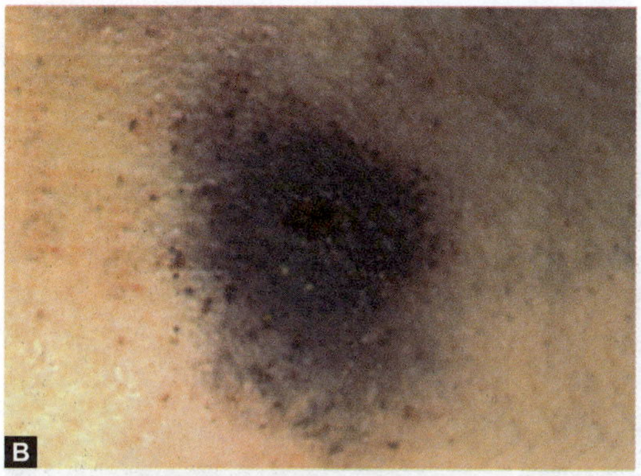

Two supporting points:

i.

ii.

Description

Inference:

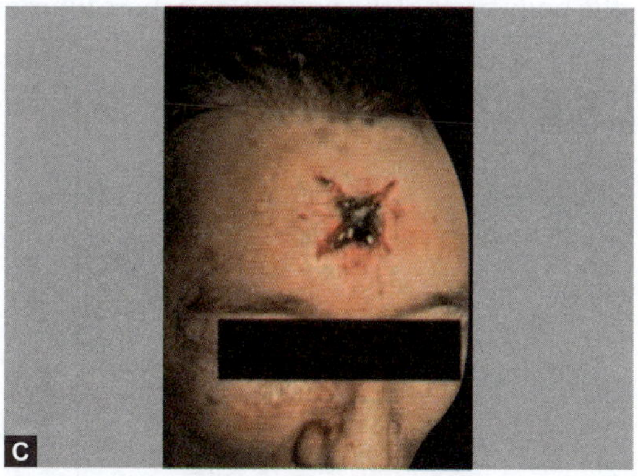

Two supporting points:

i.

ii.

Description

Inference:

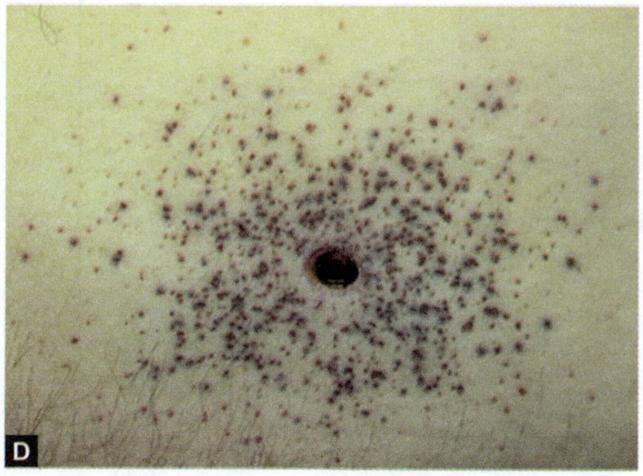

Two supporting points:

i.

ii.

11. Gunshot wound on skull causes bevelling of inner or outer table depending on whether it is entry or exit wound. Given below are two photographs of same skull in two views—one showing entry wound and another showing exit wound. Describe and identify them.
[Do mention *bevelling* to support your answer]

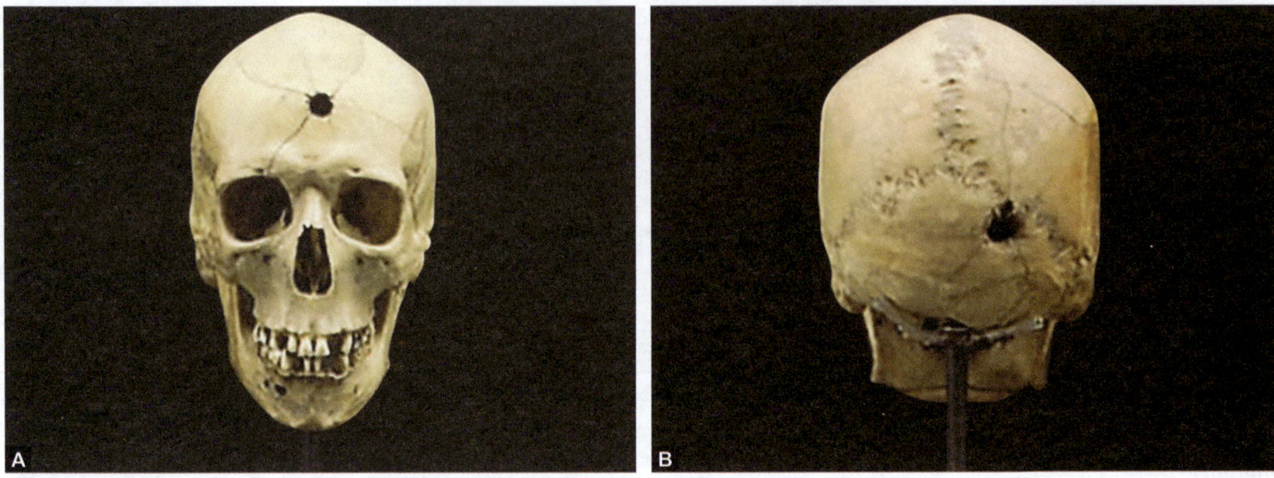

12. A schematic diagram of a road traffic accident is given below. Mention the body parts of the pedestrian, where injuries will be sustained.

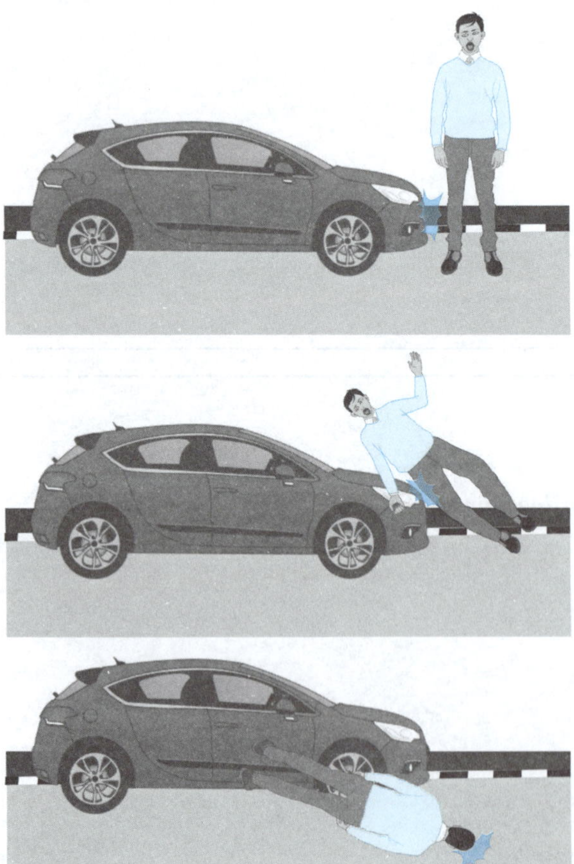

Primary impact injuries

Secondary impact injuries

Secondary injuries

13. First photo (A) is during initial impact; second photo (B) is after impact. Mention in which lobe will show coup injury and which lobe will show contrecoup injury.

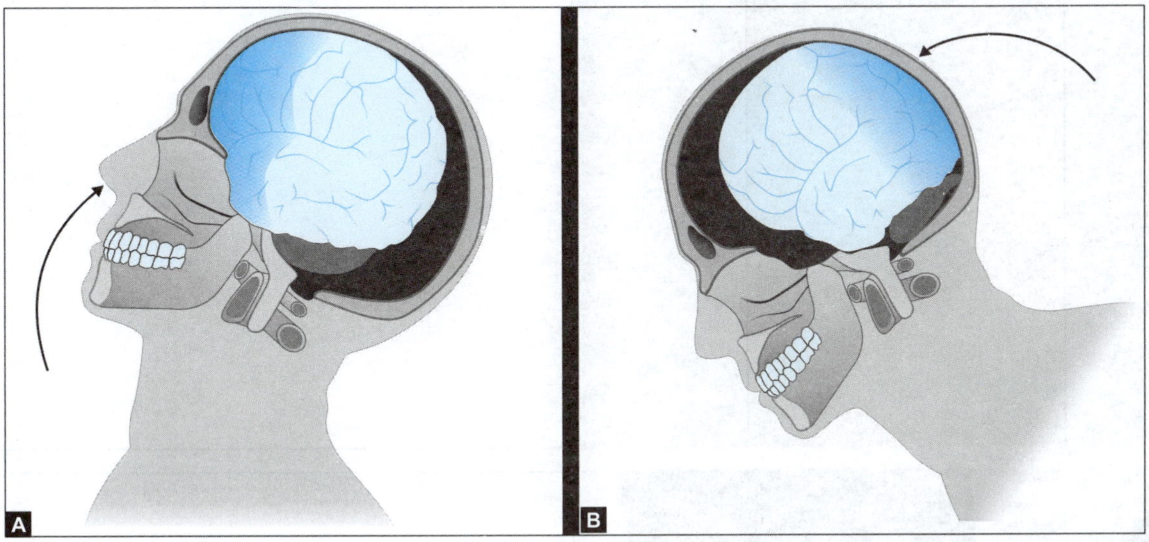

14. Describe and identify the following injuries along with the causative weapon and write their medicolegal importance.

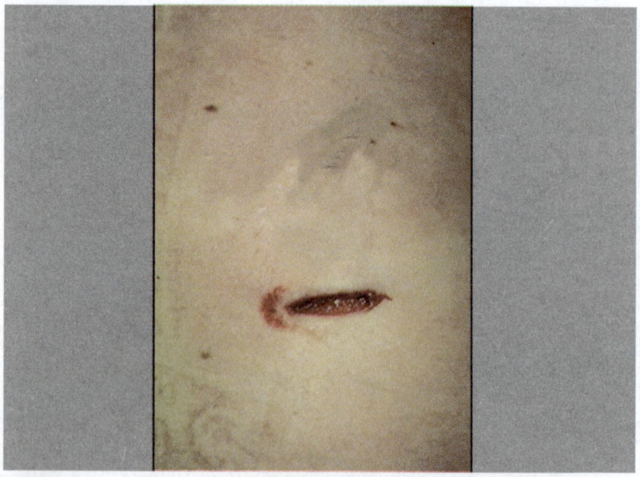

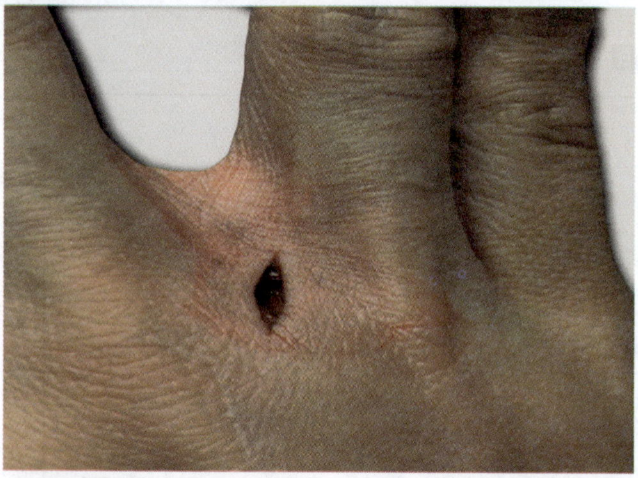

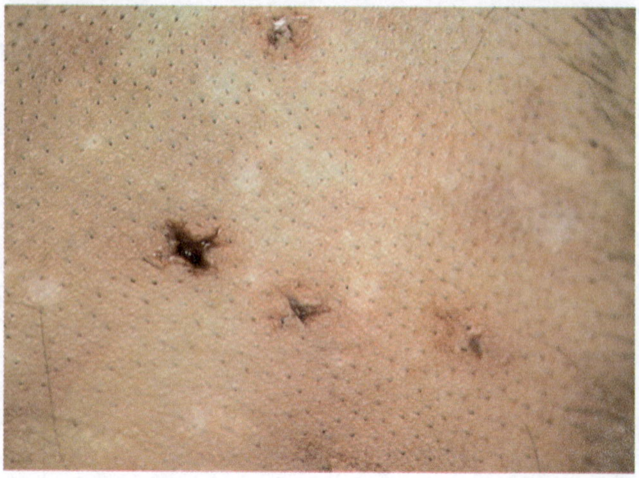

INJURY CERTIFICATE

Guideline for Writing Injury Certificate

Name of the Hospital: Name of the Department:

Reference Number:

Name of the subject: As stated by the subject, here arbitrary

Sex: As stated in the problem ***Age:*** As stated in the problem

Address: As stated by the subject, here any nearby address of your institution

Consent for examination: ***(To follow the general consent for Medicolegal Examination)***

Brought by and identified by: Self or accompanying person

Identification mark: At least two marks over exposed parts of body

Date and time of examination: Date and exact time

Date and time of occurrence
Place of occurrence } As stated by the subject or accompanying person, here as noted in the problem

History as stated by the subject or accompanying person: History of incidence in short

General examination:

Height: Measured height ***Pulse:***

Weight: Measured weight ***BP:***

Mental status: Whether alert Conscious, cooperative or not

Gait: Whether normal or not ***Condition of wearing apparel:*** Any tear or damage

Complaint of the subject: As stated by the subject, here as noted in the problem

Description of injuries:

Sl. No.	*Nature of injury*	*Site of injury*	*Size of injury*	*Simple/Grievous*	*Nature of weapon*	*Age of injury*	*Remarks*
	Which type of injury, e.g. abrasion	Which part of body it belongs as stated in the problem	Length, breadth and depth (wherever applicable)	Depending upon the clauses of grievous hurt	Blunt or sharp, heavy or light	External appearance, e.g. bluish discolouration of bruise	Any other investigation required, e.g. X-ray for suspected fracture

Treatment given: Injection Tetanus toxoid, antibiotic, etc.

Prognosis: Depending upon severity of injury

Opinion:

Date: Signature of examining doctor with Reg No.

INJURY CERTIFICATE PROBLEMS

Problem 1:

One 30-year-old male person comes to emergency department of your hospital with history of being hit by his neighbour yesterday morning at 10 am during a hot altercation in the local market. He is accompanied by his elder brother. The subject complains of pain and tenderness over right side of face. On examination, there is a bruise over right side of face over and around right malar prominence, one abrasion over posterior aspect of left elbow and adjacent part of left forearm and one small abrasion over dorsum of left hand. Write one hypothetical injury certificate and give your opinion.

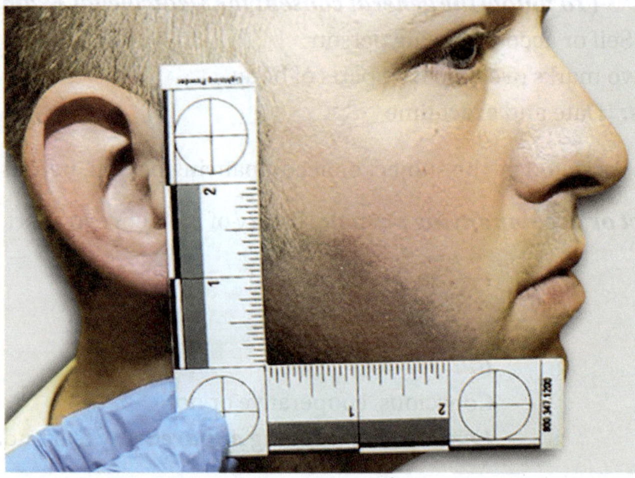

Problem 2:

One 45-year-old male person was hit by a motorcycle while walking in the road today at about 4 pm. Subsequently, he fell down on the road and received injuries on his body. He is brought to emergency department by one of his friends at about 5 pm. He presents with pain over his legs. On examination, few injuries are found over his legs, which are shown in the diagram below. Write one hypothetical injury certificate and give your opinion.

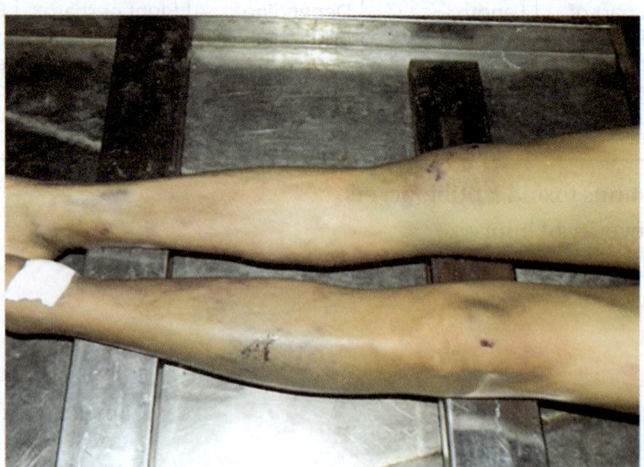

INJURY CERTIFICATE

Name of the Hospital: Name of the Department:
Reference Number:
Name of the subject:
Sex: ***Age:***
Address:
Consent for examination: ***(To follow the general consent for Medicolegal Examination)***
Brought by and identified by:
Identification mark:

Date and time of examination:
Date and time of occurrence:
Place of occurrence:
History as stated by the subject or accompanying person:

General examination:
Height: ***Pulse:***
Weight: ***BP:***
Mental status: ***Any sign of intoxication:***
Gait: ***Condition of wearing apparel:***

Complaint of the subject:

Description of injuries:

Sl. No.	*Nature of injury*	*Site of injury*	*Size of injury*	*Simple/Grievous*	*Nature of weapon*	*Age of injury*	*Remarks*

Treatment given:

Prognosis:

Opinion:

Date: Signature of examining doctor with Reg No.

INJURY CERTIFICATE

Name of the Hospital: Name of the Department:

Reference Number:

Name of the subject:

Sex: ***Age:***

Address:

Consent for examination: ***(To follow the general consent for Medicolegal Examination)***

Brought by and identified by:

Identification marks:

Date and time of examination:

Date and time of occurrence:

Place of occurrence:

History as stated by the subject or accompanying person:

General examination:

Height: ***Pulse:***

Weight: ***BP:***

Mental status: ***Any sign of intoxication:***

Gait: ***Condition of wearing apparel:***

Complaint of the subject:

Description of injuries:

Sl. No.	Nature of injury	Site of injury	Size of injury	Simple/Grievous	Nature of weapon	Age of injury	Remarks

Treatment given:

Prognosis:

Opinion:

Date: Signature of examining doctor with Reg No.

CERTIFICATE ON WEAPON EXAMINATION

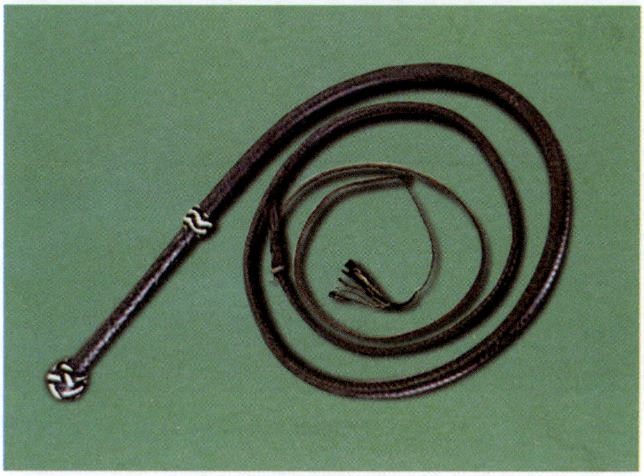

Whip

To
The IO,
.... PS,
....

Sub: Answer to the queries in connection with PS case No. 123 dated

Dear Sir,

Here is the answer to the queries respectively:

1. Report of Examination of Weapon of Offence
I am submitting here with the detailed report on examination of weapon of offence in connection with ....

Report of Examination
Date of receive:
Brought by: Mr
Date of examination:
Description

Received one sealed packet said to be the weapon of offence identified as ....

Further details are as follows:

Opinion

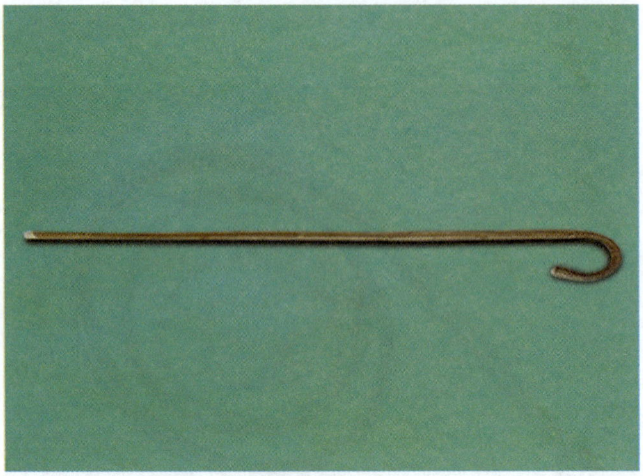

Stick

To
The IO,
.... PS,
....

Sub: Answer to the queries in connection with PS case No. 123 dated

Dear Sir,
Here is the answer to the queries respectively:

2. Report of Examination of Weapon of Offence:

I am submitting here with the detailed report on Examination of weapon of offence in connection with ....

Report of Examination

Date of receive:
Brought by: Mr
Date of examination:

Description

Received one sealed packet said to be the weapon of offence identified as ....

Further details are as follows:

Opinion

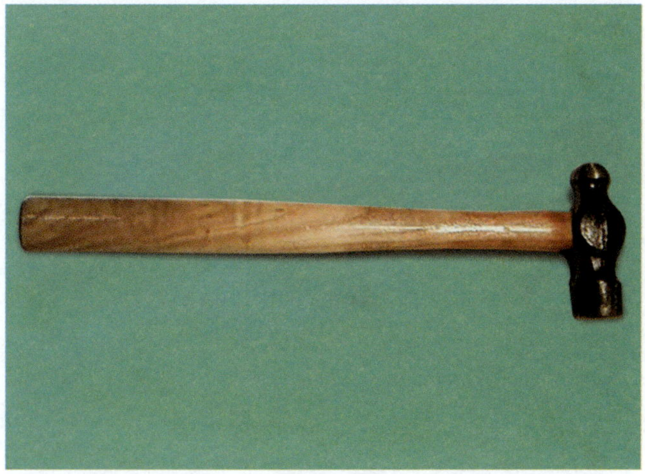

Hammer

CERTIFICATE ON WEAPON EXAMINATION

To
The IO,
.... PS,
....

Sub: Answer to the queries in connection with PS case No. 123 dated

Here is the answer to the queries respectively:

Report of Examination of Weapon of Offence

I am submitting here with the detailed report on examination of weapon of offence in connection with ....

Report of Examination
Date of receive:
Brought by: Mr
Date of examination:
Description

Received one sealed packet said to be the weapon of offence identified as ....

Further details are as follows:

Opinion

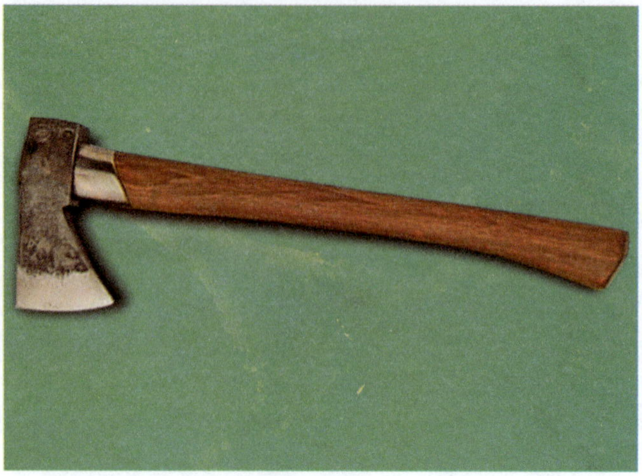

Axe

CERTIFICATE ON WEAPON EXAMINATION

To
The IO,
.... PS,
....

Sub: Answer to the queries in connection with PS case No. 123 dated

Here is the answer to the queries respectively:

Report of Examination of Weapon of Offence

I am submitting here with the detailed report on Examination of weapon of offence in connection with ....

Report of Examination

Date of receive:
Brought by: Mr
Date of examination:

Description

Received one sealed packet said to be the weapon of offence identified as ....

Further details are as follows:

Opinion

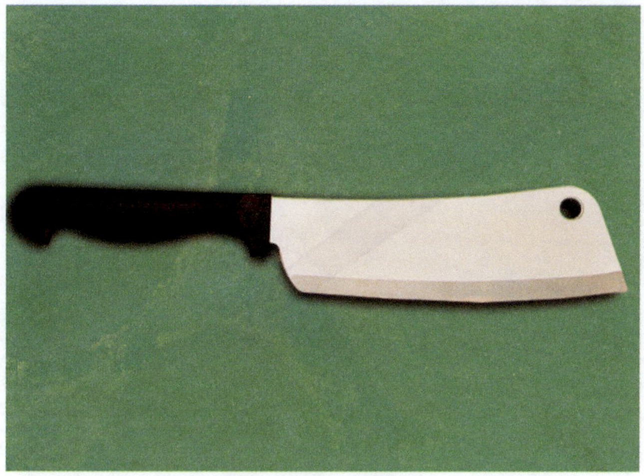

Meat chopper

CERTIFICATE ON WEAPON EXAMINATION

To
The IO,
.... PS,
....

Sub: Answer to the queries in connection with PS case No. 123 dated

Here is the answer to the queries respectively:

Report of Examination of Weapon of Offence

I am submitting here with the detailed report on examination of weapon of offence in connection with ....

Report of Examination

Date of receive:
Brought by: Mr
Date of examination:

Description

Received one sealed packet said to be the weapon of offence identified as ....

Further details are as follows:

Opinion

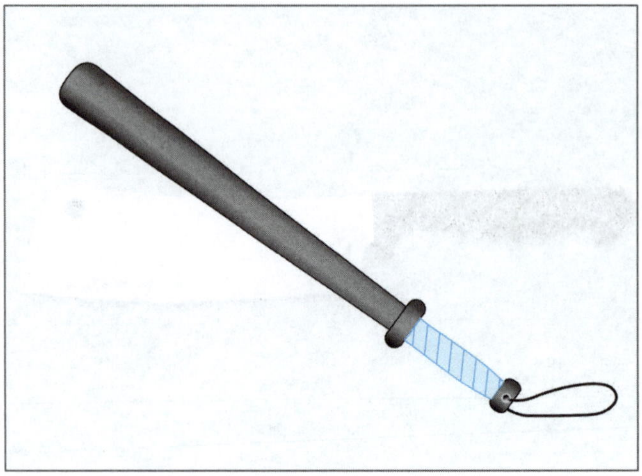

Police baton

CERTIFICATE ON WEAPON EXAMINATION

To
The IO,
.... PS,
....

Sub: Answer to the queries in connection with PS case No. 123 dated

Here is the answer to the queries respectively:

Report of Examination of Weapon of Offence

I am submitting here with the detailed report on examination of weapon of offence in connection with ....

Report of Examination
Date of receive:
Brought by: Mr
Date of examination:

Description

Received one sealed packet said to be the weapon of offence identified as ....

Further details are as follows:

Opinion

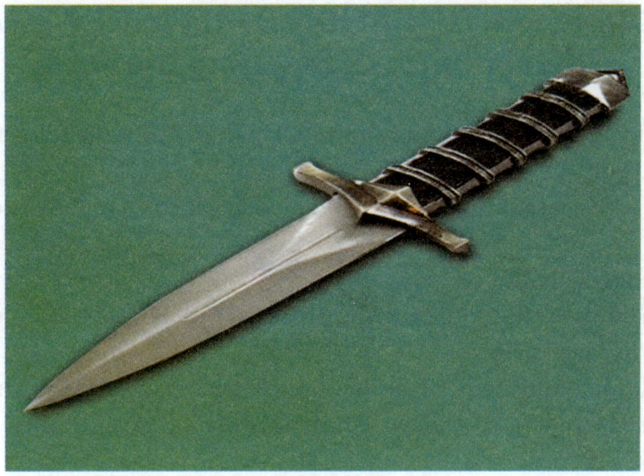

Dagger

CERTIFICATE ON WEAPON EXAMINATION

To
The IO,
.... PS,
....

Sub: Answer to the queries in connection with PS case No. 123 dated

Here is the answer to the queries respectively –

Report of Examination of Weapon of Offence

I am submitting here with the detailed report on examination of weapon of offence in connection with ....

Report of Examination
Date of receive:
Brought by: Mr
Date of examination:
Description

Received one sealed packet said to be the weapon of offence identified as ....

Further details are as follows:

i. **Length of blade:**
   Maximum breadth of the blade:
ii. **Shape:.**
iii. **Hilt:**
iv. **Handle:**

Opinion

MEDICAL CERTIFICATION OF CAUSE OF DEATH
Guidelines for Completing the Form

- **Name of the Hospital (in form 4) (not present in form 4A):** Write down the full name of the hospital along with address where the patient died.
- **Ward number (in form 4) (not present in form 4A):** Mention in which ward the patient died, e.g. MALE MEDICAL WARD-2
- Write down the **date and time of death.**
- **As noted in form 4A:** Write down the full address of the deceased with PS and also note the deceased was under your treatment from which date to which date.
- **Name of deceased:** Write down the full name of the deceased. If deceased is an infant, not yet named at time of death, mention Son of (S/O) or Daughter of (D/O), followed by names of mother and father.
- **Sex:** Male/female/third sex
- **Age:** If the deceased was over 1 year of age, give age in completed years. If the deceased was below 1 year of age, give age in months, and if below 1 month give age in completed number of days, and if below one day, in hours.
- **Cause of Death:**
  - It has 2 parts, part I (immediate cause and antecedent cause) and part II (Other significant conditions)
  - Part I is again divided into three parts, lines (a), (b), (c).
  - Immediate cause corresponds to line (a) and antecedent cause corresponds to line (b) and (c).
  - **Line (a)—IMMEDIATE CAUSE:** 'State the disease, injury or complication which caused death, not the mode of dying such as heart failure, asthenia, etc.'
    - **Explanation:** The disease or conditions directly leading to death.This does not mean the mode of dying such as heart failure, respiratory failure, cardiorespiratory failure, neurocardiorespiratory failure, etc. These terms should never appear on the certificate since these are modes of dying and not at all causes of death. Every death is associated with cardiac failure and respiratory failure, without stoppage of these three vital systems (cardiac, respiratory and nervous) no death is possible. So they are not cause of death.
    - Similarly, old age or senility should be not given as a cause of death. If old age was contributory factor, it can be mentioned in part II.
  - **Line (b)—ANTECEDENT CAUSE:** 'Morbid conditions, if any giving rise to the above cause, stating underlying conditions last'
    - **Explanation:** Next consider whether the immediate cause, mentioned in line (a) is a complication or delayed result of some other cause. If it is so, mention the antecedent cause in part I, line (b).
      An antecedent condition have just have prepared the way for the immediate cause of death, by damage to tissues or impairment of function, even after a long interval.
  - **Line (c)—ANTECEDENT CAUSE:** Consider whether the antecedent cause, mentioned in line (b) is a complication or delayed result of some other cause. If it is so, mention the antecedent cause in part I, line (c).
    If the sequence of events comprises more than three stages, extra line (and entries) may be made in part I as line (d)
    - **Note:** If a single morbid condition completely explains the deaths, rather sufficient to cause death, then it will be written on Part I line (a), and nothing more is needed to be written in the rest of Part I (line b or in line c), e.g. gastroenteritis and lobar pneumonia, are sufficient to cause death.
      However, if a number of morbid conditions were present at death, and then doctor must complete the certificate in the proper above-directed manner so that the correct underlying cause will be tabulated.

- **PART-II : OTHER SIGNIFICANT CONDITIONS**: 'Contributing to death but not related to the diseases or conditions causing it'
  - **Explanation:** These are all other diseases or conditions which were unfavourably influenced the course of the morbid process and thus contributed to the outcome but which were not related to the disease or condition directly causing death. Morbid conditions or injuries may be present which were not directly related to the chain of events causing death but which contributed in some way to the fatal outcome. For example, the patient died due to lobar pneumonia which is the immediate cause of death, but also had type 2 diabetes mellitus and hypertension. So in part II Type 2 diabetes mellitus and hypertension can be mentioned as other significant conditions but they never directly related to lobar pneumonia.
- **Interval between onset and death (approx):** Fill the column for interval between onset and death, whenever possible.
- **Manner of Death (in form 4) (not present in form 4A):**
  - Natural like lobar pneumonia, myocardial infarction, CVA, etc.
  - If the cause of death is known, but it is not known to the doctor that whether it was the result of an accident, suicide or homicide and needs further investigation, the cause of death should invariably be filled in and the manner of death should be marked as 'Pending investigation'.
- **Maternal or female deaths:** Information on pregnancy and delivery is needed in case of death of women in the child-bearing age even though the pregnancy may have had nothing to do with the death.
- **Accidental or violent deaths:** Both the cause and the nature of the injury are needed and should be stated. Like (a) Hypostatic pneumonia; (b) Fracture of neck femur; (c) Fall at bathroom, manner: Pending investigation.
- **Name and signature of the Medical Attendant certifying the cause of death and date of certification:** Put your full legible signature with date. Also write down your full name in capital letters, along your registration number with official seal.
- The form has a detachable portion separated by perforation mark, containing information on the fact of death, which after filling 4/4A will be handed over to relatives of the deceased for further procedures.

Lacunae Seen in the Certification of Cause of Death in Form No 4, Regarding Medicolegal Cases

1. In case of deaths due to violence, the column "Interval between onset and death" cannot be mentioned.
   Comment: When the death occurs after admission to the hospital, then only interval between onset and death can be mentioned.
2. In many cases, bodies are brought dead from the outside. In such cases, it is not possible to write the chain of event leading to death in form no. 4 as the past history of the patient/circumstances of injury is not known.
   Comment: In these cases, only "Immediate cause of death" can be given after post-mortem examination while antecedent cause as well as other significant conditions cannot be commented since the past history of the patient is not always known. When the cause of death is injury, specify the nature of injury (e.g. fracture, dislocation, crush injury, etc.) along with part of body involved as an immediate cause.
3. While commenting on "manner of death", it is not always possible to conclude about the exact manner of death. The reason for this is when a dead body is sent for autopsy along with inquest and dead body challan, information furnished by investigating officer is as per his inquiry. During the preliminary inquiry, he may not be able to get correct information. But from later investigations, the situation may appear to be different. In such cases, if the comment is made on manner of death on available information, then it may create problems in the court of law. Whenever possible, it can be commented but in other cases, instead of helping the judiciary, it may mislead them.
   Comment: Manner to be established by circumstantial evidences from investigation point of view.

FEW EXAMPLES WITH CASE HISTORIES

1. On 3/10/2017, a 58-year-old female was admitted with a " Strangulated Femoral Hernia" which had started 4 day earlier. She came complaining of abdominal pain and fecal vomits. Apparently, the small intestines were perforated even before. On the same day , she underwent a release of hernia and the recession of the Intestines, with an end to end "Anastomosis". On the next day, she started developing signs of "peritonitis", and following that died on 14/10/2017.
   Ans:
   Part I: Immediate cause of death:
   a. Peritonitis
   b. Perforation of small intestine
   c. Strangulated femoral hernia
   Part II ....[Kept blank]
   Explanation: It simply means strangulated femoral hernia was the triggering event which cases perforation of small intestine which leads to peritonitis causing death.
2. On 1st Feb, a 52-year-old man presented at a clinic with complaining of hemoptysis and loss of weight. On examination, he was found to be anemic, and therefore admitted in hospital. The diagnosis was made advanced pulmonary tuberculosis reactivation type with cavitations, perhaps of 8 years duration. The patient also suffered from generalized atherosclerosis probably of long duration. He also had varicose vein of lower extremities. On admission, the patient had acute and massive pulmonary hemorrhage and died that evening.
   Ans:
   Part I
   a. Acute pulmonary hemorrhage
   b. Advanced pulmonary tuberculosis reactivation type with cavitation
   Part II: Generalized atherosclerosis, varicose vein of lower extremities
3. A 69-year-old female was admitted to the hospital with shock with signs of septicemia along with gangrene of (Right) foot. Patient had swelling of right foot and fever since 3 days. She had history of chronic obstructive pulmonary disease (COPD) due to chronic bronchitis and had diabetes since 5 years. Patient had diagnosed as complications of carcinoma of pancreas and operated for the same 5 years back. Patient died 2 days after admission due to septicaemic shock.
   Ans:
   Part I: Immediate cause of death:
   a. Septicaemic shock
   b. Gangrene of right foot
   c. Diabetes mellitus
   d. Carcinoma pancreas
   Part II: COPD due to chronic bronchitis.
4. A 70-year-old female was admitted to the hospital for fracture neck femur 6 hours back due to fall in a bathroom. She was known diabetic since 10 years and hypertensive since 15 years. Open reduction of the fracture was advised but operation was delayed for fitness. On 6th day, patient deteriorated becoming severe breathless and had sudden collapse showing signs of pulmonary embolism. Patient died after 5 hours.
   Ans:
   Part I: Immediate cause of death:
   a. Pulmonary embolism
   b. Fracture neck femur
   c. Fall in bathroom
   Part II: Diabetes mellitus and hypertension.

PROBLEMS ON MCCD

1. A 21-year-old female, 2nd para, had a full-term normal delivery at home. On 7th day of puerperium, she had high-grade fever with chills though fever was neglected for another 2 days. On 9th day of puerperium patient was shifted to the hospital following deterioration of condition. On examination, patient was febrile with temperature 102 °F and had foul-smelling vaginal discharge. Further examination revealed uterus was not involuted and had tenderness over both fornices. Blood examination revealed patient had severe anaemic (Hb 3.5 g%). Patient was treated vigorously. On the same day, patient developed oliguria, hypotension with other features of acute renal failure because of puerperal sepsis. Patient died on 11th day of puerperium.

   Based on the above-noted information fill the MCCD Form.
2. A lady aged 25 years was admitted to a hospital with history of 80% dermoepidermal burn injury. Police gave the history, it was a suicidal attempt though patient party claimed that she was burnt by her in laws in relation to demand of dowry. She developed septicemia and died after 5 days of admission.
3. ***To be given by the teacher:***

FORM NO. 4

(See Rule 7)

MEDICAL CERTIFICATION OF CAUSE OF DEATH

(Hospital in-patients. Not to be used for stillbirths)

To be sent to Registrar along with Form No.2 (Death Report)

Name of the Hospital .... I hereby certify that the person whose particulars are given below died in the hospital in Ward No. .... on .... at ... AM/PM

<table>
<tr><td colspan="5">NAME OF DECEASED</td><td>For use of Statistical Office</td></tr>
<tr><td>Sex</td><td colspan="4">Age at Death</td><td></td></tr>
<tr><td></td><td>If 1 year or more age in years</td><td>If less than 1 year, age in months</td><td>If less than 1 month, age in days</td><td>If less than 1 day, age in hours</td><td rowspan="4"></td></tr>
<tr><td>1. Male
2. Female</td><td></td><td></td><td></td><td></td></tr>
<tr><td colspan="4">CAUSE OF DEATH</td><td rowspan="2">Interval between on set & death approx.</td></tr>
<tr><td colspan="2">I
Immediate cause
State the disease, injury or complication which caused death, not the mode of dying, such as heart failure, asthenia, etc.
Antecedent cause
Morbid conditions, If any, giving rise to the above cause, stating underlying conditions last

II
Other significant conditions contributing to the death but not related to the disease or conditions causing it</td><td colspan="2">(a) ....
Due to (or as a consequences of)
(b) ....
Due to (or as a consequences of)

(c) ....

....
....</td></tr>
</table>

Manner of Death: How did the injury occur?

1. Natural 2. Accident 3. Suicide 4. Homicide
5. Pending investigation

If decreased was a female, was the death associated with pregnancy? 1. Yes 2. No

If yes, was there a delivery? 1. Yes 2. No

Name and signature of the Medical Attendant certifying the cause of death

Date of certification ....

REVERSE FOR INSTRUCTIONS

(To be detached and handed over to the relative of the deceased)

Certified that Shri/Smt/Kum ....S/W/D of Shri .... R/O .... Was admitted to this hospital on .... and expired on ....

Doctor ....

(Signature with Reg No.)

FORM NO. 4A

(See Rule 7)

MEDICAL CERTIFICATION OF CAUSE OF DEATH

(For noninstitutional deaths. Not to be used for stillbirths)

To be sent to Registrar along with Form No. 2 (Death Report)

Name of the Hospital .... I hereby certify that the person whose particulars are given below died in the hospital in Ward No. .... on .... at ... AM/PM

<table>
<tr><td colspan="5">NAME OF DECEASED</td><td>For use of Statistical Office</td></tr>
<tr><td>Sex</td><td colspan="4">Age at Death</td><td></td></tr>
<tr><td></td><td>If 1 year or more age in years</td><td>If less than 1 year, age in months</td><td>If less than 1 month, age in days</td><td>If less than 1 day, age in hours</td><td rowspan="4"></td></tr>
<tr><td>1. Male
2. Female</td><td></td><td></td><td></td><td></td></tr>
<tr><td colspan="4">CAUSE OF DEATH</td><td rowspan="2">Interval between on set & death approx.</td></tr>
<tr><td colspan="2">I
Immediate cause
State the disease, injury or complication which caused death, not the mode of dying, such as heart failure, asthenia, etc.
Antecedent cause
Morbid conditions, If any, giving rise to the above cause, stating underlying conditions last

II
Other significant conditions contributing to the death but not related to the disease or conditions causing it</td><td colspan="2">(a) ....
Due to (or as a consequences of)
(b) ....
Due to (or as a consequences of)

(c) ....

....
..................</td></tr>
</table>

Manner of Death

How did the injury occur?

1. Natural 2. Accident 3. Suicide 4. Homicide

5. Pending investigation

If deceased was a female, was the death associated with pregnancy? 1. Yes 2. No

If yes, was there a delivery? 1. Yes 2. No

Name and signature of the Medical Attendant certifying the cause of death

Date of certification ....

REVERSE FOR INSTRUCTIONS

(To be detached and handed over to the relative of the deceased)

Certified that Shri/Smt/Kum .... S/W/D of Shri .... R/O .... Was admitted to this hospital on .... and expired on ....

Doctor ....

(Signature with Reg No.)

FORM NO. 4A

(See Rule 7)

MEDICAL CERTIFICATION OF CAUSE OF DEATH

(For noninstitutional deaths. Not to be used for stillbirths)

To be sent to Registrar along with Form No. 2 (Death Report)

Name of the Hospital .... I hereby certify that the deceased Shri/Smt/Kum ....son of/wife of/daughter of.. resident of .... was under my treatment from .... to .... and he/she died on .... at ....AM/PM

<table>
<tr><td colspan="5">NAME OF DECEASED</td><td>For use of Statistical Office</td></tr>
<tr><td>Sex</td><td colspan="4">Age at Death</td><td></td></tr>
<tr><td></td><td>If 1 year or more age in years</td><td>If less than 1 year, age in months</td><td>If less than 1 month, age in days</td><td>If less than 1 day, age in hours</td><td rowspan="4"></td></tr>
<tr><td>1. Male
2. Female</td><td></td><td></td><td></td><td></td></tr>
<tr><td colspan="4">CAUSE OF DEATH</td><td rowspan="2">Interval between on set & death approx.</td></tr>
<tr><td colspan="2">I
Immediate cause
State the disease, injury or complication which caused death, not the mode of dying, such as heart failure, asthenia, etc.
Antecedent cause
Morbid conditions, If any, giving rise to the above cause, stating underlying conditions last

II
Other significant conditions contributing to the death but not related to the disease or conditions causing it</td><td colspan="2">(a) ....
Due to (or as a consequences of)
(b) ....
Due to (or as a consequences of)

(c) ....
....
....</td></tr>
</table>

If decreased was a female, was the death associated with pregnancy? 1. Yes 2. No

If yes, was there a delivery? 1. Yes 2. No

Name and signature of the Medical Practitioner certifying the cause of death

Date of certification ....

REVERSE FOR INSTRUCTIONS

(To be detached and handed over to the relative of the deceased)

Certified that Shri/Smt/Kum ....S/W/D of Shri .... R/O .... Was under my treatment from .... to .... and he/she expired on .... at .... AM/PM.

Doctor ....

(Name of Doctor)

FORM OF CERTIFICATE RECOMMENDED FOR LEAVE OR EXTENSION OR COMMUNICATION OF LEAVE

[MCI: Code of Medical Ethics, Regulation 2002]

Signature of patient or thumb impression ....

(To be filled up by the applicant in the presence of the Government Medical Attendant, or Medical Practitioner.)
Identification marks:

1. ....

2. ....

I, Dr .... after careful examination of the case certify

hereby that .... whose signature is given above is

suffering from .... and I consider that a period of absence from duty of ......

.... with effect from .... is absolutely necessary for the restoration of his health.

Place ....

Date ....

Signature of

Registered Medical Practitioner

Registration No. ....

(Medical Council of India/State Medical Council of .... State)

Note: The nature and probable duration of the illness should also be specified. This certificate must be accompanied by a brief resume of the case giving the nature of the illness, its symptoms, causes and duration.

FORM OF CERTIFICATE RECOMMENDED FOR FITNESS [MCI: Code of Medical Ethics, Regulation 2002]

Signature of patient or thumb impression ....

(To be filled up by the applicant in the presence of the Government Medical Attendant, or Medical Practitioner.)

Identification marks:

1. ....

2. ....

I, Dr .... certify hereby that Mr/Mrs/Miss ....

.... whose signature is given above was suffering from ....

.... and was advised for ....

Now, after careful examination of the case, I certify hereby that he/she on restoration of health is now fit to join service.

Place ....

Date ....

Signature of

Registered Medical Practitioner

Registration No. ....

(Medical Council of India/State Medical Council of .... State)

Note: The nature and probable duration of the illness should also be specified. This certificate must be accompanied by a brief resume of the case giving the nature of the illness, its symptoms, causes and duration.

SICKNESS–FITNESS PROBLEMS

1. Ms Sonali met an accident on 20/09/2017 and suffered acute swelling and pain over left foot. On X-ray of left foot, nondisplaced fracture of 4th metatarsal bone was seen. You put a plaster of Paris (POP) cast for immobilization and asked her to take rest with limited mobility for 3 weeks. Write down a sickness as well as fitness certificate for her.
2. Mr Abhishek Dutta came to you on 21/09/2017 with complain of fever for last 2 days along with cough, tachypnea and respiratory distress. On examination, rhonchi was present, decreased intensity of breath sound, dullness on percussion were found. Laboratory investigation shows elevated total leukocyte count, dyselectrolytemia with homogenous consolidation on chest X-ray. He was being treated under your care. Write down a sickness certificate for Mr Dutta allowing him a week of leave as well as issue a fitness certificate after his complete recovery.
3. ***To be given by the teacher.***

DYING DECLARATION

I, Dr...Son/Daughter of.., working as ...., residing at ...., in presence of witnesses (1) ....Son/Daughter of... residing at.. and (2)..Son/Daughter of.. residing at .... shall record the dying declaration of .... male/female aged ......years, S/o ....residing at ....at..am/pm, on (date) ...., at (place) .... in the word by word order as narrated by the declarant.

Before recording this dying declaration, I have examined the declarant and found that his/her condition is in a possession of a mind to deliver and he/she may die any time hereafter, in spite of the life-saving treatment being given to him/her. I have also thoroughly examined his/her level of consciousness, orientation of time and space, memory and other mental faculties, and I hereby certify that the declarant is in possession of a sound mind to deliver his dying declaration. The words of the declarant as said by him are ....
....
....
....
....

In order to clarify the points as revealed by the answers to the questions recorded in continuation to this, I asked the following questions to which the declarant gave the answers, which are recorded in that sequence

Question:..
....

Answer:..
....
....

I, Dr ....certify that the above declaration was recorded by me and I also certify that the declarant ....maintained his/her sound state of mind throughout the dictation of his/her declaration. The recording ended at ....am/pm on ....

Pulse: ..../min. **BP: ....mm of Hg.**

Signature:

Name & Address of the Medical Practitioner

Read over to me and found to be correct

(Should be translated into declarant's mother tongue)

Recorded and signed in my presence

Signature, Name &
Address of First Witness:

Signature, Name &
Address of Second Witness:

Signature:

Name & Address of the Declarant:

Date.............................

CERTIFICATE OF DRUNKENNESS

Requisition received from the ....
of .... police station, dated ....
for the examination and certification of drunkenness of ....
.... aged .... years and accompanied by HC/PC No. ....
Name: .... Age: ....years. Sex: Male/Female.
Address: ....
....
Consent: ....

Whether under arrest or not (to be specified in requisition): Yes/No
Date & time of arrest (as specified in the requisition): ....
Date & time of examination: ....
Identification marks:
1. ....
2. ....
History:
a. Relevant to consumption of alcohol: ....
b. Relevant to illness, if any: ....
Smell of alcohol in breath: Present/Absent.
General appearance & behavior:
 a. Clothing : Decently dressed/Disordered/Soiled/Torn.
 b. General disposition : Calm/Talkative/Abusive/Aggressive.
 c. Speech : Normal/Thick and slurred/incoherent.
Eyes: (a) Conjunctiva: Normal/Congested. (b) Pupils: Normal/Dilated/Sluggishly reacting.
Higher functions:
 (a) Self control: Normal/Impaired. (b) Memory: Normal/Impaired.
 (c) Orientation of time & space: Normal/Impaired. (d) Reaction time: Normal/Delayed.
Muscular co-ordination:
 (a) Gait: Normal/Unsteady/Unable to stand upright.
 (b) Finger nose test: Positive/Negative.
Systemic examination findings:
Pulse: ..../min. BP : ....mm of Hg. Reflexes: Normal/Exaggerated/Sluggish.
Romberg's sign: Positive/Negative.
Any other findings/Injuries on the body: ....

Smell of alcohol in breath : Persisting/Not persisting.
Special examination (Blood & Urine) : Preserved/Not preserved.

Opinion:

1. **There is nothing on examination to suggest that the person has consumed alcohol.**
2. **The person examined has consumed alcohol, but is not under the influence of alcohol.**
3. **The person examined has consumed alcohol and is under the influence of alcohol.**

Date: .... Signature: ....
Place: .... Name: ....
Name of Institution:
.... Designation : ....
(Strike off which is not applicable)
Received the certificate: .... (Signature & PC No.)

Date:........................

CERTIFICATE OF EXAMINATION BY A MEDICAL OFFICER

As per requisition from...
dated......................, physical examination of ....
S/o..., (address)..
....,
involved in crime number...of .... police station
was done at...am/pm on......................... at ....
Consent:...
....

Identification marks:

1. ....
2. ....

History (Related to illness/injury, if any):
....
....

Findings of physical examination:

A. *General:* *Height:* ....cm. *Weight:* ....kg. Build & nourishment: Poor/Moderate/Obese.
Pallor: Present/Absent. Physical deformity, if any: ....
Others if any: ....

B. Systemic examination: Pulse: ..../min. Blood pressure: ....mm of Hg.
CVS, NS, RS & GIS: ....
....

C. Injuries (If any): ....
....
....
....
....
....

D. Investigations, if any: ....

Opinion:

There is no evidence of any clinically identifiable illness.
There are no injuries on the person/injuries on the person could be caused as alleged.**
Suggestions, if any :...

Date: .... Signature: ....
Place: .... Name: ....
Name of Institution:
.... Designation: ....
(Strike off which is not applicable)
Received the certificate : .... (Signature & PC No.)

MEDICAL EXAMINATION REPORT OF AN ACCUSED OF SEXUAL ASSAULT (GUIDELINES FOR REPORT WRITING)

***Ref*:** As provided in the problem
Date and time of examination:
Name of the subject: As provided in the requisition, here arbitrary
Stated age: As provided in the problem
Brought and identified by: Name and designation of the police personnel, here arbitrary
Examination in presence of: Name and designation of the attendant, here arbitrary
Identification mark: 1.
2.

General examination:
Height: Measured height, here arbitrary
Weight: Measured height, here arbitrary
Mental status: Sound, alert, co-operative
Gait: Normal
Voice: Developed as per age

Scalp hair:
Axillary hair:
Beard:
Moustache:
Pubic hair:
} Length, color, appearance

Tooth: Number of tooth, permanent or temporary, spacing present or not, attrition present or not

Genital examination:
Penis: Length and mid shaft circumference in flaccid condition and on manipulation.

Testes and scrotum: Whether healthy or having any abnormality or disease or injury
Foreskin: Whether healthy or not
Urethral discharge: Present or not, amount, if present
Smegma: Present or not which is related with time passed since last sex act
Anus: Whether healthy or having any abnormality or disease or injury
Any injury around genitalia: Present or not

Any injury over any other body part: Present or not

Any disease or deformity: Present or not on naked eye examination
Materials preserved: Name of the articles preserved and purpose of preservation

Opinion: 1.Whether capable of performing sexual intercourse depending upon findings of genital examination. 2. Whether any clinical evidence of venereal disease and final opinion by chemical examination report of urethral swab and smear. 3. Give your opinion depending upon presence or absence of vaginal epithelial cells in urethral swab and smear.

Signature of Doctor

PROBLEMS ON MEDICAL EXAMINATION OF AN ACCUSED OF SEXUAL ASSAULT

Problem 1.

One 19-year-old girl complains to police that she has been subjected to forceful sexual intercourse 18 hours back by one 30 years old man who was a stranger to the girl. One case has been filed with ref Bowbazar PS Case No. 335 dated 12.10.2017 u/s 376 IPC. One suspected accused person has been arrested by the police 6 hours back who has confessed the crime. The person has been produced to you for medical examination and on examination you noticed one small scratch abrasion over right side of the face and three small scratch abrasions over dorsum of right hand. No injury around genitalia detected. Write down one hypothetical report of medical examination of the suspected accused person providing your opinion on the following points:

i. Whether the person is able to perform sexual intercourse?
ii. Whether the person is suffering from any venereal disease?
iii. Whether the person has performed any sexual intercourse in recent past?

Problem 2.

One 25-year-old girl complaint to police that one 35 years old man who is known to her performed sexual intercourse with her several times by imposing on her a false belief of marriage. On the basis of the complain, one case has been filed with ref ABC PS Case No. 552 dated 28.9.2017 u/s 376 IPC. The accused person has been arrested by police and brought to you for medical examination. On examination, no injury could be detected over any body part of the person including genitalia. Write down one hypothetical report of medical examination of the suspected accused person providing your opinion on the following points:

i. Whether the person is able to perform sexual intercourse?
ii. Whether the person is suffering from any venereal disease?
iii. Whether the person has performed any sexual intercourse in recent past?

Problem 3

To be given by teachers.

MEDICAL EXAMINATION REPORT OF AN ACCUSED OF SEXUAL ASSAULT

Ref:
Date and time of examination:
Name of the subject:
Stated age:
Brought and identified by:
Examination in presence of:
Identification marks: 1.

2.

General examination:

Height:	***Scalp hair:***
Weight:	***Axillary hair:***
Mental status:	***Beard:***
Gait:	***Moustache:***
Voice:	***Pubic hair:***
Tooth:	

RIGHT	LEFT

GENITAL EXAMINATION

Penis:

Testes and scrotum:

Foreskin:

Frenulum:

Urethral discharge:

Smegma:

Anus:

Any injury around genitalia:

Any injury over any other body part:

Any disease or deformity:

Radiological examination, if required:

Materials preserved:

Opinion:

Signature of Doctor

MEDICAL EXAMINATION REPORT OF AN ACCUSED OF SEXUAL ASSAULT

Ref:
Date and time of examination:
Name of the subject:
Stated age:
Brought and identified by:
Examination in presence of:
Identification marks: 1.

2.

General examination:

Height:
Weight:
Mental status:
Gait:
Voice:
Teeth:

Scalp hair:
Axillary hair:
Beard:
Moustache:
Pubic hair:

RIGHT	LEFT

GENITAL EXAMINATION

Penis:

Testes and scrotum:

Foreskin:

Frenulum:

Urethral discharge:

Smegma:

Anus:

Any injury around genitalia:

Any injury over any other body part:

Any disease or deformity:

Radiological examination, if required:

Materials preserved:

Opinion:

Signature of Doctor

MEDICAL EXAMINATION REPORT OF A VICTIM/SURVIVOR OF SEXUAL ASSAULT (GUIDELINES FOR REPORT WRITING)

Guideline for writing medical examination report of A Victim girl of sexual assault:

NAME OF THE DOCTOR
DESIGNATION: DATE: ***Date of examination*** AT: ***Time of examination***
REF: as provided in requisition
NAME: ***Name of the girl in capital letter,*** STATED AGE: ***As stated in the requisition***
BROUGHT BY: ***Name and designation of the police officer by whom brought and identified***
POLICE STATION: ***Name of the police station***
NAME AND DESIGNATION OF FEMALE ATTENDANT DURING EXAMINATION:
....

MARKS OF IDENTIFICATION: ***At least two permanent identification marks in respect to their nature, location and distance from fixed bony prominences***

When the victim girl cannot sign

Thumb Impression

SIGNATURE: Signature of the victim girl
NAME: Name of the victim girl
DATE: Date of examination

PHYSICAL EXAMINATION: ***FEMALE***

1. HEIGHT: ***Measured in cm/ft and inches***
2. WEIGHT: ***Measured weight in KGS***
3. GENERAL BUILT: GOOD/AVERAGE/POOR } ***As noticed during examination***
4. BEHAVIOUR: SOBER/ECCENTRIC/ERRATIC } ***As noticed during examination***
5. SIGN OF DRUNKENNESS: ***Present/Absent***
6. GAIT: ***Normal/Any abnormality seen***
7. INTELLIGENCE:
8. HAIR: ***Length, color and appearance*** (i) AXILLARY:(ii) PUBIC: (iii) SCALP HAIR:
9. TEETH:

RIGHT	LEFT

10. ABDOMEN: Pain and tenderness present or not; soft or rigid
11. BREAST: (i) DEVELOPMENT: ***As noticed on examination, here as per age*** (ii) AREOLA: ......***color***...... (iii) NIPPLES: ....***as per age***
12. DEVELOPMENT OF THE GENITALIA: ***WELL DEVELOPED/PRE-PUBERTAL***
13. LABIA MAJORA: ***Sign of inflammation, any injury, whether apposed or not***
14. LABIA MINORA: ***Sign of inflammation, injury***

15. STATEMENT OF THE PERSON BEING EXAMINED: ***As history given by the subject, here arbitrary.***
    INCIDENCE OCCURRED ON .... AT ABOUT .... AM/PM, AT ....AREA
    POSITION OF THE VICTIM DURING THE ACT: STANDING/LYING ON GROUND
    MENSTRUAL HISTORY DURING THE ACT: AMENORRHEA/MENSTRUATING. LMP ....
    STATUS OF SENSORIUM DURING THE ACT: IN FULL SENSE/INTOXICATED
    AFTER THE ACT, WHETHER SHE:
    CHANGED CLOTHING: YES/NO, AT .... AM/PM ON ....
    TOOK BATH: YES/NO, AT .... AM/PM ON ....
    PASSED URINE: YES/NO, AT .... AM/PM ON ....
    PASSED MOTION: YES/NO, AT .... AM/PM ON ....
16. EXAMINATION OF THE CLOTHING WORN AT THE TIME OF THE ACT: ***Stain present or not, any tear or damage***
    STAIN OF: ***BLOOD/SEMEN/OTHER DISCHARGE/MUD & DIRT***
17. GENITAL AREA:
    PUBIC HAIR: MATTED/NOT MATTED
    VISIBLE EXTERNAL SIGNS OF INJURY AT: ***Injury present or not, if present describe each injury in relation to their nature, colour***

VULVA:	YES/NO	DESCRIPTION --
HYMEN:	YES/NO	DESCRIPTION --
FOURCHETTE:	YES/NO	DESCRIPTION --
PERINEUM:	YES/NO	DESCRIPTION --
VAGINA:	YES/NO	DESCRIPTION --
CERVIX:	YES/NO	DESCRIPTION --

18. VISIBLE EXTERNAL SIGNS OF INJURY ON THE BODY OTHER THAN GENITALIA: ***Present or not, if present write in details***
19. X-RAY EXAMINATION ADVISED: YES/NO indicated when age of the girl is to be determined
20. X-RAY TAKEN ON:
21. X-RAY FINDING:
22. SMEAR (S) COLLECTED FROM: ***As per requirement of the particular case.***

VAGINA:	YES/NO	FOR SPERMATOZOA & SMEGMA BACILLUS/**DNA** PROFILE
URETHRA:	YES/NO	FOR ....
ORAL CAVITY:	YES/NO	FOR ....
ANUS:	YES/NO	FOR ....

23. BLOOD SAMPLE COLLECTED: YES/NO, FOR: GROUPING AND X–MATCHING/**DNA** PROFILE
    SMEAR (S) &/or BLOOD SAMPLE DULY SEALED AND PACKED, HANDED OVER TO:
    .... OF .... PS

24. ANY OTHER TESTS DONE:
    URINE FOR B-hCG: YES/NO, RESULT
    TEST FOR HIV: YES/NO,

25. OPINION:

Genital injuries	*Physical injuries*	*Opinion*	*Rationale why forced penetrative sex cannot be ruled out*	*What can FSL detect?*
Present	Present	There are signs suggestive of recent use of force/forceful penetration of vagina/anus. Sexual violence cannot be rules out	Evidence for semen and spermatozoa are yet to be tested by laboratory examinations in case of penile penetration	Evidence of semen except when condom was used
Present	Absent	There are signs suggestive of recent forceful penetration of vagina/anus	Evidence for semen and spermatozoa are yet to be tested in case of penile penetration. The lack of physical injuries could be because of the survivor being unconscious, under the effect of alcohol/drugs, overpowered or threatened. It could be because, there was fingering or penetration by object with or without use of lubricant, which is an offence under Sec 375 IPC	Evidence of semen or lubricant except when condom was used
Absent	Present	There are signs of use of force, however vaginal or anal or oral penetration cannot be ruled out	The lack of injuries could be because of the survivor being unconscious, under the effect of alcohol/drugs, overpowered or threatened or use of lubricant	Evidence of semen or lubricant
Absent	Absent	There are no signs of use of force; however, final opinion is reserved pending availability of FSL reports. Sexual violence cannot be ruled out	The lack of genital injuries could be because of use of lubricant. The lack of physical injuries could be because of the survivor being unconscious, under the effect of alcohol/drugs, overpowered or threatened. It could also be because, there was fingering or penetration by object with use of lubricant, which is an offence under Sec 375 IPC	Evidence of semen, lubricant and drug/alcohol

26. FINAL OPINION: To be formulated after receiving reports from the FSL

Sl. No.	Genital	Physical injuries/ diseases	FSL report injuries/diseases	Final opinion
For penile penetration				
1.	Present	Present	Positive for presence of semen	There are signs suggestive of forceful vaginal/ anal intercourse
2.	Present	Absent	Positive for presence of semen	There are signs suggestive of forceful vaginal/ anal intercourse
3.	Absent	Present	Positive for presence of semen	There are signs suggestive of forceful vaginal/ anal intercourse
4.	Absent	Absent	Positive for presence of semen	There are signs suggestive of vaginal/anal intercourse
5.	Absent	Absent	Positive for drugs/alcohol and semen	There are signs suggestive of vagina/anal intercourse under the influence of drugs/alcohol
For non-penile penetration				
6.	Present	Present	FSL report is negative for presence of semen/ alcohol/drugs/lubricant	There are no signs suggestive of vaginal/anal intercourse, but there is evidence of physical and genital assault
7.	Present	Absent	FSL report is negative for presence of semen/ alcohol/drugs/lubricant	There are no signs suggestive of vaginal/anal intercourse, but there is evidence of genital assault
8.	Absent	Present	FSL report is negative for presence of semen/ alcohol/drugs/lubricant	There are no signs suggestive of vagina/anal intercourse, but there is evidence of physical assault
9.	Absent	Absent	FSL report is negative for presence of semen/ alcohol/drugs/lubricant	There are no signs suggestive of penetration of vaginal/anal
10.	Absent	Absent	FSL report is positive for presence of lubricant only	There is a possibility of vaginal/anal penetration by lubricated object

PROBLEMS ON MEDICAL EXAMINATION OF A VICTIM OF SEXUAL ASSAULT

Problem 1.

One 19-year-old girl complaint to police that she has been subjected to forceful sexual intercourse 18 hours back by one 30-year-old man who was a stranger to the girl. One case has been filed with ref Bowbazar PS Case No 335 dated 12.10.2017 u/s 376 IPC. The girl has been produced to you for medical examination and on examination you noticed signs of inflammation around vulva, bruise over labia, tears over posterior margin of hymen and small scratch abrasions over inner aspect of thigh and breast. Write down one hypothetical report of medical examination of the victim girl providing your opinion on the following point:

Whether the girl has been subjected to recent forceful sexual intercourse?

Problem 2.

One 30-year-old lady complaint to police that one 35-year-old man who is known to her performed sexual intercourse with her several times by imposing on her a false belief of marriage. On the basis of the complain, one case has been filed with ref ABC PS Case No 552 dated 28.9.2017 u/s 376 IPC. The lady has been brought to you by police for medical examination. On examination, no recent injury could be detected over any body part of the lady including genitalia. Write down one hypothetical report of medical examination of the victim girl providing your opinion on the following points:

i. Whether the lady has been subjected to recent sexual intercourse?
ii. Whether she is suffering from any venereal disease?

Problem 3.

To be given by the teacher.

CONFIDENTIAL

DEPARTMENT OF FORENSIC MEDICINE AND TOXICOLOGY

____________________ MEDICAL COLLEGE

MEDICOLEGAL CERTIFICATE FOR FEMALE

NAME OF THE DOCTOR:
DESIGNATION: DATE: AT:
REF:
NAME: STATED AGE:
BROUGHT BY: SIGNATURE:
POLICE STATION:
NAME AND DESIGNATION OF FEMALE ATTENDANT DURING EXAMINATION:
MARKS OF IDENTIFICATION: 1.

2.

CONSENT FOR MEDICAL EXAMINATION: (TAKEN SEPARATELY)

SIGNATURE:
NAME:
DATE:

Thumb Impression

PHYSICAL EXAMINATION: FEMALE

1. HEIGHT:
2. WEIGHT: Kg
3. GENERAL BUILT: GOOD/AVERAGE/POOR
4. BEHAVIOUR: SOBER/ECCENTRIC/ERRATIC
5. SIGN OF DRUNKENNESS:
6. GAIT:
7. INTELLIGENCE:
8. HAIR: (i) AXILLARY: (ii) PUBIC: (iii) SCALP HAIR:
9. TEETH:

RIGHT	LEFT

10. ABDOMEN:
11. BREAST: (i) DEVELOPMENT: (ii) AREOLA: .... (iii) NIPPLES: ....
12. DEVELOPMENT OF THE GENITALIA: WELL DEVELOPED/PREPUBERTAL

13. LABIA MAJORA:
14. LABIA MINORA:
15. STATEMENT OF THE PERSON BEING EXAMINED:
    INCIDENCE OCCURRED ON .... AT ABOUT .... AM/PM, AT .... AREA
    POSITION OF THE VICTIM DURING THE ACT: STANDING/LYING ON GROUND
    MENSTRUAL HISTORY DURING THE ACT: AMENORRHEA/MENSTRUATING. LMP ....
    STATUS OF SENSORIUM DURING THE ACT: IN FULL SENSE/INTOXICATED
    AFTER THE ACT, WHETHER SHE:
    CHANGED CLOTHING: YES/NO, AT .... AM/PM ON ....
    TOOK BATH: YES/NO, AT .... AM/PM ON ....
    PASSED URINE: YES/NO, AT .... AM/PM ON ....
    PASSED MOTION: YES/NO, AT .... AM/PM ON ....
16. EXAMINATION OF THE CLOTHING WORN AT THE TIME OF THE ACT:
    STAIN OF: BLOOD/SEMEN/OTHER DISCHARGE/MUD AND DIRT
17. GENITAL AREA:
    PUBIC HAIR: MATTED/NOT MATTED
    VISIBLE EXTERNAL SIGNS OF INJURY AT:
    VULVA: YES/NO DESCRIPTION ....
    HYMEN: YES/NO DESCRIPTION ....
    FOURCHETTE: YES/NO DESCRIPTION ....
    PERINEUM: YES/NO DESCRIPTION ....
    VAGINA: YES/NO DESCRIPTION ....
    CERVIX: YES/NO DESCRIPTION ....
18. VISIBLE EXTERNAL SIGNS OF INJURY ON THE BODY OTHER THAN GENITALIA.
19. X-RAY EXAMINATION ADVISED: YES/NO
20. X-RAY TAKEN ON:
21. X-RAY FINDING:

22. SMEAR (S) COLLECTED FROM:
    VAGINA: YES/NO FOR SPERMATOZOA AND SMEGMA BACILLUS/DNA PROFILE
    URETHRA: YES/NO FOR ....
    ORAL CAVITY: YES/NO FOR ....
    ANUS: YES/NO FOR ....
23. BLOOD SAMPLE COLLECTED: YES/NO, FOR: GROUPING AND X–MATCHING/DNA PROFILE
    SMEAR (S) &/OR BLOOD SAMPLE DULY SEALED AND PACKED, HANDED OVER TO:
    .... OF .... PS
24. ANY OTHER TESTS DONE:
    URINE FOR B-hCG: YES/NO, RESULT
    TEST FOR HIV: YES/NO,
25. OPINION:

PROF/ASSOC PROF/ASSTT PROF/DEMONSTRATOR
DEPARTMENT OF FORENSIC MEDICINE & TOXICOLOGY
____________________ MEDICAL COLLEGE
WEST BENGAL

DEPARTMENT OF FORENSIC MEDICINE AND TOXICOLOGY

____________________ MEDICAL COLLEGE

MEDICOLEGAL CERTIFICATE FOR FEMALE

NAME OF THE DOCTOR:
DESIGNATION: DATE: AT:
REF:
NAME: STATED AGE:
BROUGHT BY: SIGNATURE:
POLICE STATION:
NAME AND DESIGNATION OF FEMALE ATTENDANT DURING EXAMINATION:
MARKS OF IDENTIFICATION: 1.

2.

CONSENT FOR MEDICAL EXAMINATION: (TAKEN SEPARATELY)

SIGNATURE:
NAME:
DATE:

Thumb Impression

PHYSICAL EXAMINATION: FEMALE

1. HEIGHT:
2. WEIGHT: Kg
3. GENERAL BUILT: GOOD/AVERAGE/POOR.
4. BEHAVIOUR: SOBER/ECCENTRIC/ERRATIC.
5. SIGN OF DRUNKENNESS:
6. GAIT:
7. INTELLIGENCE:
8. HAIR: (i) AXILLARY: (ii) PUBIC: (iii) SCALP HAIR:
9. TEETH:

RIGHT	LEFT

10. ABDOMEN:
11. BREAST: (i) DEVELOPMENT: .... (ii) AREOLA: .... (iii) NIPPLES: ....
12. DEVELOPMENT OF THE GENITALIA: WELL DEVELOPED/PRE-PUBERTAL

13. LABIA MAJORA:
14. LABIA MINORA:
15. STATEMENT OF THE PERSON BEING EXAMINED:
    INCIDENCE OCCURRED ON .... AT ABOUT .... AM/PM, AT .... AREA
    POSITION OF THE VICTIM DURING THE ACT: STANDING/LYING ON GROUND
    MENSTRUAL HISTORY DURING THE ACT: AMENORRHEA/MENSTRUATING. LMP ....
    STATUS OF SENSORIUM DURING THE ACT: IN FULL SENSE/INTOXICATED
    AFTER THE ACT, WHETHER SHE:
    CHANGED CLOTHING: YES/NO, AT .... AM/PM ON ....
    TOOK BATH: YES/NO, AT .... AM/PM ON ....
    PASSED URINE: YES/NO, AT .... AM/PM ON ....
    PASSED MOTION: YES/NO, AT .... AM/PM ON ....
16. EXAMINATION OF THE CLOTHING WORN AT THE TIME OF THE ACT:
    STAIN OF: BLOOD/SEMEN/OTHER DISCHARGE/MUD & DIRT
17. GENITAL AREA:
    PUBIC HAIR: MATTED/NOT MATTED
    VISIBLE EXTERNAL SIGNS OF INJURY AT:
    VULVA: YES/NO DESCRIPTION ....
    HYMEN: YES/NO DESCRIPTION ....
    FOURCHETTE: YES/NO DESCRIPTION ....
    PERINEUM: YES/NO DESCRIPTION ....
    VAGINA: YES/NO DESCRIPTION ....
    CERVIX: YES/NO DESCRIPTION ....
18. VISIBLE EXTERNAL SIGNS OF INJURY ON THE BODY OTHER THAN GENITALIA.
19. X RAY EXAMINATION ADVISED: YES/NO
20. X-RAY TAKEN ON:
21. X-RAY FINDING:

22. SMEAR (S) COLLECTED FROM:
    VAGINA: YES/NO FOR SPERMATOZOA AND SMEGMA BACILLUS/DNA PROFILE
    URETHRA: YES/NO FOR ....
    ORAL CAVITY: YES/NO FOR ....
    ANUS: YES/NO FOR ....
23. BLOOD SAMPLE COLLECTED: YES/NO, FOR: GROUPING AND X–MATCHING/DNA PROFILE
    SMEAR (S) AND/OR BLOOD SAMPLE DULY SEALED AND PACKED, HANDED OVER TO:
    .... OF .... PS
24. ANY OTHER TESTS DONE:
    URINE FOR β-hCG: YES/NO, RESULT
    TEST FOR HIV: YES/NO,
25. OPINION:

PROF/ASSOC PROF/ASSTT PROF/DEMONSTRATOR
DEPARTMENT OF FORENSIC MEDICINE & TOXICOLOGY
____________________ MEDICAL COLLEGE
WEST BENGAL

DEPARTMENT OF FORENSIC MEDICINE AND TOXICOLOGY

____________________ MEDICAL COLLEGE

MEDICOLEGAL CERTIFICATE FOR FEMALE

NAME OF THE DOCTOR:
DESIGNATION: DATE: AT:
REF:
NAME: STATED AGE:
BROUGHT BY: SIGNATURE:
POLICE STATION:
NAME AND DESIGNATION OF FEMALE ATTENDANT DURING EXAMINATION:
MARKS OF IDENTIFICATION: 1.

2.

CONSENT FOR MEDICAL EXAMINATION: (TAKEN SEPARATELY)

SIGNATURE:
NAME:
DATE:

Thumb Impression

PHYSICAL EXAMINATION: FEMALE

1. HEIGHT:
2. WEIGHT: Kg
3. GENERAL BUILT: GOOD/AVERAGE/POOR.
4. BEHAVIOUR: SOBER/ECCENTRIC/ERRATIC.
5. SIGN OF DRUNKENNESS:
6. GAIT:
7. INTELLIGENCE:
8. HAIR: (i) AXILLARY: (ii) PUBIC: (iii) SCALP HAIR:
9. TEETH:

RIGHT LEFT

10. ABDOMEN:
11. BREAST: (i) DEVELOPMENT: .... (ii) AREOLA: .... (iii) NIPPLES: ....
12. DEVELOPMENT OF THE GENITALIA: WELL DEVELOPED/PRE-PUBERTAL

13. LABIA MAJORA:
14. LABIA MINORA:
15. STATEMENT OF THE PERSON BEING EXAMINED:
    INCIDENCE OCCURRED ON .... AT ABOUT .... AM/PM, AT .... AREA
    POSITION OF THE VICTIM DURING THE ACT: STANDING/LYING ON GROUND
    MENSTRUAL HISTORY DURING THE ACT: AMENORRHEA/MENSTRUATING. LMP ....
    STATUS OF SENSORIUM DURING THE ACT: IN FULL SENSE/INTOXICATED
    AFTER THE ACT, WHETHER SHE:
    CHANGED CLOTHING: YES/NO, AT .... AM/PM ON ....
    TOOKBATH: YES/NO, AT .... AM/PM ON ....
    PASSED URINE: YES/NO, AT .... AM/PM ON ....
    PASSED MOTION: YES/NO, AT .... AM/PM ON ....
16. EXAMINATION OF THE CLOTHING WORN AT THE TIME OF THE ACT:
    STAIN OF: BLOOD/SEMEN/OTHER DISCHARGE/MUD & DIRT
17. GENITAL AREA:
    PUBIC HAIR: MATTED/NOT MATTED
    VISIBLE EXTERNAL SIGNS OF INJURY AT:
    VULVA: YES/NO DESCRIPTION ....
    HYMEN: YES/NO DESCRIPTION ....
    FOURCHETTE: YES/NO DESCRIPTION ....
    PERINEUM: YES/NO DESCRIPTION ....
    VAGINA: YES/NO DESCRIPTION ....
    CERVIX: YES/NO DESCRIPTION ....
18. VISIBLE EXTERNAL SIGNS OF INJURY ON THE BODY OTHER THAN GENITALIA.
19. X RAY EXAMINATION ADVISED: YES/NO
20. X-RAY TAKEN ON:
21. X-RAY FINDING:

22. SMEAR (S) COLLECTED FROM:
    VAGINA: YES/NO FOR SPERMATOZOA AND SMEGMA BACILLUS/DNA PROFILE
    URETHRA: YES/NO FOR ....
    ORAL CAVITY: YES/NO FOR ....
    ANUS: YES/NO FOR ....
23. BLOOD SAMPLE COLLECTED: YES/NO, FOR: GROUPING AND X–MATCHING/DNA PROFILE
    SMEAR (S) AND/OR BLOOD SAMPLE DULY SEALED AND PACKED, HANDED OVER TO:
    .... OF .... PS
24. ANY OTHER TESTS DONE:
    URINE FOR β-hCG: YES/NO, RESULT
    TEST FOR HIV: YES/NO,
25. OPINION:

PROF/ASSOC PROF/ASSTT PROF/DEMONSTRATOR
DEPARTMENT OF FORENSIC MEDICINE & TOXICOLOGY
____________________ MEDICAL COLLEGE
WEST BENGAL

Identify the Kit and Write its Different Parts

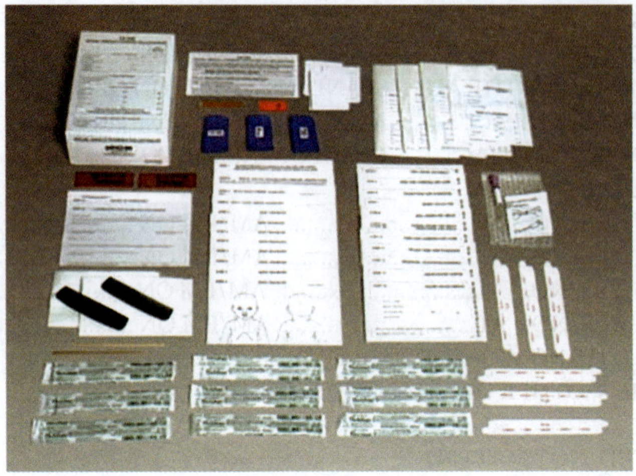

CONSENT
INFORMED CONSENT FORM FOR MEDICOLEGAL EXAMINATION

Name of the Hospital: ....

Name of the Department: FORENSIC MEDICINE AND TOXICOLOGY

Date & Time:

Reference:

Name of the subject:

Sex: Stated age:

Name of the legal guardian from whom consent is obtained, if subject cannot give a valid consent and also state the reason why consent is obtained from legal guardian:

Name and designation of the witness under whose presence the consent is obtained:

Name of the interpreter/special educator, if applicable:

....

....

DECLARATION BY THE SUBJECT/LEGAL GUARDIAN

I...hereby give my consent freely, willingly, voluntarily without any force or coercion for medicolegal examination and necessary specimen collection which includes the followings:

1. My/his/her rights of informed refusal before or any time during examination and possible consequences of such refusal for medicolegal examination.
2. The purpose and possible outcome of this examination.
3. The result of this examination will be supplied to the concerned authority under whose direction or request this examination is being conducted and the same report may be used in Court in future.
4. Noting the history of the case for which my/his/her examination is being done.
5. Noting the identification marks from which I/he/she can be identified later on.
6. Full undressing before the doctor and attendant, if required.
7. Taking photographs, if required for evidential purpose and the same may be supplied to the concerned authority under whose direction or request this examination is being conducted and the same may be produced before Court.
8. The data collected during examination can be used for academic purpose and can be kept as a part of hospital records keeping my/his/her identity anonymous.
9. A through physical examination including examination of external genitalia, dental examination and radiological examination, if deemed fit so by the examining doctor.
10. Collection of specimens which includes wearing apparels, nail cuttings and scrapings, pubic hairs, plucked out tuft of scalp hairs, blood, saliva, semen, urethral swab. Swab may be taken from any area over my/his/her body as deemed fit by the examining doctor, swab from vulva, vagina, cervix, perineum, medial aspects of thighs, swab may be taken from glans penis, corona glands, anus, mouth. Whatever applicable to me/him/her for the interest of the case.

11. The collected specimens will be forwarded to the concerned authority for necessary examination and will be treated as per legal norms.
12. I/he/she may be referred to other specialty for further examination, if required.
13. I acknowledge that the examining doctor has answered my specific queries and concerns about this examination.
14. Being a male/female, I have no objection for undergoing examination before a male/female doctor and his/her attendant.
15. I certify and acknowledge that I have read this consent form carefully taking my time/it has been explained properly to me in the language clearly understood by me and that language is ....
16. I am hereby authorizing the doctor to conduct my/his/her medicolegal examination and necessary sample collection as deemed necessary.

....

Full signature/thumb impression of the subject/legal guardian/the person in whom the subject reposes trust giving consent with date.

....

Full signature of the witness with date

....

....

INTERPRETER'S/SPECIAL EDUCATOR'S DECLARATION (IF APPLICABLE)

I .... confirm that I have accurately interpreted the contents of this form and related conversation between the doctor and the subject/the person consenting on behalf of the subject.

....

Full signature of the interpreter/special educator with date

....

Full signature of the witness with date

DECLARATION BY THE EXAMINING DOCTOR

I declare that I have explained the purpose, procedure, possible outcome of the medicolegal examination and informed refusal with its consequences to the subject identified as.../the person consenting on behalf of the subject named../the interpreter or special educator named..

I have given the subject/the person consenting on behalf of the subject all opportunities to ask questions related to the examination and I have answered these questions from my best knowledge and intention.

....

Full signature of the doctor with date and official seal
Registration number:
Designation:

CONSENT FORM FOR APPENDICECTOMY

Name of the Hospital:
Med Rec No.....................................
Surname...
Forename...
Date of Birth.....................................
PROPOSED TREATMENT

The doctor has explained that I *(name of patient)* .... the undersigned/ my patient... (Am) suffering from/may have/has appendicitis and for that an **Appendicectomy** is proposed.
This means removing the appendix surgically.

Under a general anaesthetic, the surgeon makes a short cut in the lower right side of the abdomen, through the skin and muscles. The appendix can be tucked behind the bowel, and sometimes the wound must be lengthened to retrieve it safely. The blood vessels to the appendix and the base of the appendix are tied off, and the appendix is removed. The operation site is checked for bleeding and the areais washed out.

If the appendix is normal, it is still removed, but the surgeon carefully checks nearby organs such as the small bowel and, in women, the ovary for other possible causes of the symptoms.

The wound is closed with absorbable sutures that do not need to be removed.

Antibiotics are usually given, especially, if the appendix is inflamed to reduce the risks of infection.

RISKS

These are the commoner risks. There may be other unusual risks that have not been listed here. Please ask your surgeon if you have any concerns.
I understand there are risks associated with any **anaesthetic** (see separate Anaesthetic Consent Form).
I/my patient may have side effects from any of the drugs used. The commoner side effects include light-headedness, nausea, skin rash and diarrhoea or constipation.
I understand an **Appendicectomy** has the following **specific risks and limitations**:

- Wound may become infected, becoming red painful, swollen and possibly developing a discharge. I/my patient may need antibiotics, if this happens.
- The surgeon may remove a normal appendix as there is no absolutely reliable test to diagnose appendicitis. Even if the appendix is apparently normal, it will still be removed.
- In some patients, other problems are encountered which may need treatment at the time, such as a bleeding ovarian cyst, or a growth on the bowel. Sometimes, this requires a different operation or a larger wound. It may happen in this case also.
- If the appendix has already ruptured, there is a real risk of an abscess developing after the operation. This usually responds to intravenous antibiotics, but sometimes requires further drainage. If the surgeon thinks this is likely, (s) he may place a drain (a small plastic tube) at the operation site. This comes out through the skin and remains in place for a few days.

- After any abdominal surgery, scar tissue can form inside the abdomen. Loops of bowel can become twisted and blocked as a result. This can happen at any time, from soon after surgery to many years later. If it happens, the blockage will require treatment in hospital. Sometimes another operation is necessary to unblock the bowel.

I understand some of the above risks are more likely if I (my patient) smoke, am overweight, diabetic, have high blood pressure or have had previous heart disease.

INDIVIDUAL RISKS

I understand the following are possible significant **risks and complications specific to my/my patient's individual circumstances** that may affect my decision to agree to have the proposed treatment:

....

....

....

DECLARATION BY PATIENT

- **I acknowledge that the surgeon has informed me about the procedure, any alternative treatments like conservative treatment, pros and cons about the alternative treatment and the proposed treatment, cost, risks, advantages of both treatments and answered my specific queries and concerns about this matter and after understanding clearly, I agreed for proposed appendicectomy willingly and the doctor has maintained my autonomy.**
- I acknowledge that I have discussed with the surgeon any significant risks and complications **specific to my/my patient's individual circumstances** that may affect my decision to agree to have an Appendicectomy.
- I agree to the disposal by the hospital authorities of any tissues that may be removed during the procedure. I understand some tissues or samples may be kept as part of my hospital records.
- I agree to any **additional procedures** considered necessary in the judgment of the surgeon during this operation.
- I understand that a doctor other than the specialist surgeon may perform the procedure.
- I have received a copy of this form to take home with me.
- I certify and acknowledge that I have read this form carefully/it has been explained to me in language clearly understood by me, that I understood the risks, alternatives explained to me.
- I am giving my Consent without any compulsion, freely and willingly and hereby authorizing the staff of the department of surgery to provide surgical service as deemed necessary.

Signature of patient **Date:** ....

Signature of the person consenting, if patient not ....

Relationship with patient: .... **Date:** ....

DECLARATION BY DOCTOR

I declare that I have respected the patient's autonomy regarding selection of proposed treatment and its alternatives and explained the nature of surgery to be performed and discussed the risks that particularly concern patient/the person consenting on behalf of the patient.

I have given the patient/the person consenting on behalf of the patient an opportunity to ask question and I have answered these to my level best.

Doctor's Signature .... **Date:** ....

INTERPRETER'S DECLARATION

I confirm that I have accurately interpreted the contents of this form and related conversation between the doctor and the patient/the person consenting on behalf of the patient.

Interpreter's name ....

Interpreter's signature.. **Date:**................................

Witness: .... **Date:**................................

CONSENT FORM FOR LAPAROSCOPIC CHOLECYSTECTOMY

Name of the Hospital:
PROPOSED TREATMENT
The doctor has explained that I, (name of patient) ...., have gallstones in my gallbladder and that a laparoscopic cholecystectomy is proposed:

This means removing the gall bladder, using a telescopic camera and instruments to avoid a large abdominal wound. Under a general anaesthetic, the abdomen is inflated with carbon dioxide gas to create a space for the surgeon to work. The surgeon sees what he/she is doing using a small telescopic camera, inserted through a small cut near the umbilicus ("belly button"). Other instruments are inserted through separate small cuts in the abdomen.

The gallbladder is carefully freed from its connections to the liver and the duct from the gallbladder to the gut is cleared. An X-ray is then taken to ensure the ducts are clear of stones and to check the anatomy. Clips are put across the cystic duct to close it off and the duct is cut. The blood supply to the gallbladder is dealt with in the same way.

The gallbladder may be emptied, if necessary and it is then removed through one of the cuts. If small stones are found in the common bile duct, these will be removed, if possible.

As much gas as possible is sucked out, the instruments are removed and the cuts are closed with stitches and/or Steri-strips. A small suction tube drain may be left in the operation area to remove any secretions.

RISKS

These are the commoner risks. There may be other unusual risks that have not been listed here. Please ask your general surgeon, if you have any general or specific concerns.

I understand there are risks associated with any anaesthetic (see separate Anaesthetic Consent Form).

I may have side effects from any of the drugs used. The commoner side effects include light-headedness, nausea, skin rash and constipation. There is a rare risk of a reaction to the X- ray dye used to examine the ducts.

I understand the procedure has the following general risks and limitations of laparoscopic surgery:

- It may be necessary to convert to an open operation because of technical difficulties or for reasons of safety.
- After the operation, I may feel nauseated, feel some shoulder-tip pain and/or abdominal bloating or pain.
- I may have some bleeding, which may rarely require a second operation or possibly a blood transfusion.
- My wounds may become infected causing redness, increased pain and discharge. I may need antibiotics.
- Damage to my bowel, bladder and blood vessels may occur due to the technique itself. If this happens, I will need open surgery to correct the damage. Very rarely, if this damage is not recognised at the time of surgery, later surgery will be necessary.
- I may develop a clot in my legs (deep vein thrombosis), causing pain and swelling and part of this may come loose and travel to my lungs (pulmonary embolus). This may make me short of breath, and occasionally may even be fatal.
- I may develop areas of minor collapse in the lungs, increasing my risk of getting a chest infection. I may need treatment with physiotherapy.
- I may have a heart attack from strain on my heart or a stroke.

I understand the procedure has the following **specific risks and limitations:**

- Important structures including the main bile duct and the main artery to the liver lie close to the gallbladder and may be injured during the operation. This will usually be repaired at the time of the operation, but may sometimes require further surgery later.
- Bile may leak from the operation site. This will usually stop spontaneously, but may require a further procedure to drain any collections or occasionally to deal with the cause.

- Rarely, other abdominal organs may be inadvertently injured during the operation and require repair, usually at the same time.

I understand the above risks are more likely if I smoke, am overweight, diabetic, have high blood pressure or have had previous heart disease.

INDIVIDUAL RISKS

I understand the following are possible significant risks and complications specific to my individual circumstances, that I have considered in deciding to have this operation:

....

....

DECLARATION BY PATIENT

- **I acknowledge the general surgeon has informed me about the procedure, alternative treatments such as conservative medical management, open cholecystectomy, pros and cons about the alternative treatments and the proposed treatment, cost, risks, advantages of all treatments, duration of hospital stay and answered my specific queries and concerns about this matter and after understanding clearly I agreed for proposed laparoscopic cholecystectomy surgery willingly and the doctor has maintained my autonomy.**
- **I acknowledge that I have discussed with the general surgeon any significant risks and complications specific to my individual circumstances that I have considered in deciding to have this operation.**
- **I agree to any other additional procedures considered necessary in the judgement of my general surgeon during this operation.**
- **I consent to a blood transfusion, if needed (patient to circle and initial choice) YES/NO**
- **I agree to the disposal by the hospital authorities of any tissues that may be removed during the procedure. I understand that some tissues or samples may be kept as part of my hospital records.**
- **I understand that a doctor other than the specialist general surgeon may perform the procedure.**
- **I have received a copy of this form to take home with me.**
- **If any staff member is exposed to my blood (needlestick injury), then I consent to a sample of my blood being collected for testing for infectious diseases, such as Hepatitis B, C and HIV. I understand that I will be counselled as soon as practicable afterwards, if this has been necessary.**
- **I am giving my consent without any compulsion, freely and willingly and hereby authorizing the staff of the department of surgery to provide surgical service as deemed necessary.**

Signature of patient **Date: ....**

Signature of the person consenting, if patient not ....

Relationship with patient: .... Date: ....

DECLARATION BY DOCTOR

I declare that I have respected the patient's autonomy regarding selection of proposed treatment and its alternatives, advantages and disadvantages of all treatments and explained the nature of surgery to be performed and discussed the risks that particularly concern patient/the person consenting on behalf of the patient.

- I have given the patient/the person consenting on behalf of the patient an opportunity to ask question and I have answered these to my level best.

Doctor's Signature... **Date: ....**

INTERPRETER'S DECLARATION

I confirm that I have accurately interpreted the contents of this form and related conversation between the doctor and the patient/the person consenting on behalf of the patient.

Interpreter's name ....

Interpreter's signature... **Date:** ....

Witness: .... **Date:** ....

CONSENT FORM FOR ABDOMINOPERINEAL RESECTION

Name of the Hospital:
PROPOSED TREATMENT

The doctor has explained that I *(name of patient)* .... the undersigned/my patient.. (Am) suffering from .... for that an **abdominoperineal** resection is proposed.

This means an operation to remove the rectum and anus with creation of a colostomy (a bag on the abdominal wall). Team of surgeons may work simultaneously or one operator may work alone.

Under a general anaesthetic, a urinary catheter is placed in the bladder and the patient positioned for access to the abdomen and pelvis. The surgeon opens the abdomen and examines the extent of the disease. The attachments of the lower bowel are cut and the bowel in the pelvis is freed, while protecting other nearby structures, especially the ureters (tubes from the kidneys to the bladder). The surgeon cuts around the anus and frees the lower back passage, working upwards to meet the abdominal operation.

When the bowel is free, it is clamped at a suitable place and cut and the specimen is sent for detailed examination. The surgeon brings the cut end of the bowel out onto the abdominal wall through a separate cut to make a colostomy and stitches this into place. Tube drains may be left in the operation site and the abdominal wound is closed. Bleeding points in the pelvis are sealed and the perineal wound is closed, using one or more soft drains to reduce fluid collections. If the pelvic tissues cannot be satisfactorily closed, the area may be packed and the perineal defect will then gradually close spontaneously.

RISKS

The following are the commoner risks. There may be other unusual risks that have not been listed here. Please ask your doctor, if you have any general or specific concerns.

I understand there are risks associated with any **anaesthetic** *(see separate Anaesthetic Consent Form).*

I/my patient may have side effects from any of the drugs used. The commoner side effects include light-headedness, nausea, skin rash and constipation.

I understand the procedure has the following **general risks and limitations**:

- I/my patient may develop a clot in a leg vein (deep vein thrombosis), causing pain and swelling. Part of this may break free and move to my lungs (pulmonary embolus), making me breathless. There is a small risk I/my patient could die.
- I/my patient may develop areas of minor collapse in the lungs, increasing the risk of getting a chest infection. It may require treatment with physiotherapy.
- I/my patient may have a heart attack from strain on the heart.

I understand the procedure has the following **specific risks and limitations**:

- Bowel may not function temporarily after the operation and I/my patient will not be able to eat or drink normally until its activity returns in a few days
- Structures near the operation site, including the ureters (tubes from the kidneys to the bladder), bladder and vagina may be damaged and require repair.
- I/my patient may not be able to pass urine spontaneously for some days and in some cases may need a urinary catheter for several weeks.
- Damage to the pelvic nerves may result in sexual problems, especially for men who may have difficulty with erections or ejaculation.

- Wounds may become infected and this may delay healing and may require antibiotics.
- The colostomy may be too tight or too loose (causing a prolapse of the bowel or a hernia around the colostomy) and these may require revision.
- Loops of bowel may become stuck to the operation site (adhesions), causing blockages that may require further surgery. This can occur even years later.
- I/my patient may develop a weakness in the wounds (incisional hernia) that may require later treatment.
- The disease may recur.

I understand some of the above risks are more likely if I (my patient) smoke, am overweight, diabetic, have high blood pressure or have had previous heart disease.

INDIVIDUAL RISKS

I understand the following are possible significant **risks and complications specific to my/my patient's individual circumstances** that may affect my decision to agree to have the proposed treatment:

....

....

....

DECLARATION BY PATIENT

I acknowledge that the surgeon has informed me about the procedure, any alternative treatments such as conservative treatment, pros and cons about the alternative treatment and the proposed treatment, cost, risks, advantages of both treatments and answered my specific queries and concerns about this matter and after understanding clearly I agreed for proposed surgery willingly and the doctor has maintained my autonomy.

I acknowledge that I have discussed with the surgeon any significant risks and complications **specific to my/my patient's individual circumstances** that I have considered in deciding to have this operation.

I agree to the disposal by the hospital authorities of any tissues that may be removed during the procedure. I understand some tissues or samples may be kept as part of my hospital records.

I agree to any **additional procedures** considered necessary in the judgment of the surgeon during this operation.

I understand that a doctor other than the specialist surgeon may perform the procedure.

I consent to a **blood transfusion,** if needed *(patient to circle and initial choice) YES/NO*

I have received a copy of this form to take home with me.

I certify and acknowledge that I have read this form carefully/it has been explained to me in language clearly understood by me, that I understood the risks, alternatives explained to me.

I am giving my Consent without any compulsion, freely and willingly and hereby authorizing the staff of the department of surgery to provide surgical service as deemed necessary.

Signature of patient: **Date: ....**

Signature of the person consenting, if patient not ....

Relationship with patient: .... **Date:** ....

DECLARATION BY DOCTOR

I declare that I have respected the patient's autonomy regarding selection of proposed treatment and its alternatives and explained the nature of surgery to be performed and discussed the risks that particularly concern patient/the person consenting on behalf of the patient.

I have given the patient/the person consenting on behalf of the patient an opportunity to ask question and I have answered these to my level best.

Doctor's Signature... **Date: ....**

INTERPRETER'S DECLARATION

I confirm that I have accurately interpreted the contents of this form and related conversation between the doctor and the patient/the person consenting on behalf of the patient.

Interpreter's name ....

Interpreter's signature... **Date**: ....

Witness: .... **Date**: ....

CONSENT FORM FOR GENERAL ANAESTHESIA ± REGIONAL ANAESTHESIA (FOR MAJOR SURGERY)

Name of the Hospital:

Surname...

Forename...

Date of Birth.....................................

PROPOSED TREATMENT

The doctor has explained that I *(name of patient)* ...., the undersigned/my patient...................................... Require (s)..................................... operative procedure and for that **general and/regional anaesthesia** is proposed.

General anaesthesia involves rendering a patient unconscious before an operation. This ensures the patient is not aware of events and does not feel pain during the operation. It is produced by drugs given through a vein and/or breathed from an anaesthesia machine.

Regional anaesthesia involves using a local anaesthetic to numb a specific area of the body for surgery. Prolonged pain relief without numbness can be achieved by infusing weak solutions of local anaesthetics and narcotic drugs to particular parts of the body after surgery or injury.

Anaesthesia affects the patient's breathing and circulation, while the operation itself also causes changes to the patient's body. The anaesthetist uses special skills and equipment to monitor and manage the patient, to ensure their safety during anaesthesia and the operation.

RISKS

Death or permanent disability related to anaesthesia is rare.

Common risks for ALL patients include:

- Bruising at the site of injections or drips
- Nausea or vomiting (although the anaesthetist will limit or prevent this as far as possible)
- Sore throat from the gases and/or the breathing tube. You may notice temporary difficulty in speaking. This should improve after some hours
- Temporary muscle pains
- Temporary headache or blurred vision

Uncommon risks for ALL patients include:

- Awareness of activity in the operating room during anaesthesia, particularly during certain operations and in some emergency situations.
- Eye abrasions causing pain and requiring treatment with medication and patching.
- Damage to teeth or dental work, iips or tongue.

Extremely rare risks for ALL patients: These may cause brain damage or death and include:

- Obstructions in the breathing passages that cannot be readily controlled. These can lead to severe difficulty with breathing
- Allergy to drugs causing wheezing and rash and in rare cases, severe swelling, low blood pressure and poor circulation
- Inherited muscle sensitivity to particular anaesthetic drugs (malignant hyperthermia). This can cause a rapid rise in temperature, heart rate and breathing with high blood pressure and muscle rigidity, and
- Heart attacks, strokes and pneumonia. While these are uncommon, the risks are higher for patients with diseases of the arteries or lungs and in smokers.

Regional anaesthesia has some of the risks listed above and several other risks or consequences:

- Muscle weakness in the anaesthetized limb, or difficulty passing urine for a lower body block, while the—Anaesthetic is working.
- While this returns to normal as the drugs' effects wear off, a temporary urinary catheter may be necessary.
- Headache, which is usually short-lived but can be severe and last some days.
- Damage to nearby blood vessels or organs, e.g. lungs.
- Backache may follow spinal or epidural anaesthesia. This usually improves quickly, but occasionally can be lasting.
- There is a very small risk of infection or bleeding at the injection site, which may require antibiotic or surgical treatment.
- Rarely, nerves may be damaged resulting in long-term weakness, pain, altered sensation or paralysis.

Note: There may be other unusual risks that have not been listed here. Please ask your anaesthetist, if you have any general or specific concerns.**

I understand some of the above risks may be more likely if I (my patient) smoke, am overweight, diabetic, have high blood pressure or have had previous heart disease.

INDIVIDUAL RISKS (to be completed by the anaesthetist completing this form)
The following are examples of possible risks and complications specific to this patient:

....

....

....

Location and circumstances of obtaining this patient's consent for anaesthesia:

DECLARATION BY PATIENT/GUARDIAN/PROXY

I acknowledge the anaesthetist has informed me about the anaesthetic procedure, alternative treatments and answered my specific queries and concerns about this matter.

I acknowledge that I have discussed with the anaesthetist regarding significant risks and complications **specific to my/ my patient's individual circumstances** that I have considered in deciding to have general anaesthesia.

I understand that the type(s) of an anaesthetic service will be used for my/patient's procedure and that anaesthetic technique to be used is determined by many factors including my/patient's physical conditions, the type of procedure is to do, his or her preference, as well as my/patient's own desire.

I understand that an anaesthetist other than the consultant anaesthetist or doctor training to be a specialist anaesthetist may administer the anaesthetic.

I certify and acknowledge that I have read this form carefully/it has been explained to me in language clearly understood by me, that I understood the risks, alternatives explained to me and have been made that anaesthesia may cause unexpected complications.

I have received a copy of this form to take home with me.

I am giving my Consent without any compulsion, freely and willingly and also hereby authorizing the staff of the department of anesthesiology to provide anaesthesia service as deemed necessary.

Signature of patient **Date: ....**

Signature of the person consenting, if patient not ....

Relationship with patient: .... **Date:** ....

DECLARATION BY DOCTOR

I declare that I have explained the nature of general and/or regional anaesthesia to be given and discussed the risks that particularly concern patient/the person consenting on behalf of the patient.

I have given the patient/the person consenting on behalf of the patient an opportunity to ask question and I have answered these to my level best.

Doctor's signature... **Date:** ....

INTERPRETER'S DECLARATION

I confirm that I have accurately interpreted the contents of this form and related conversation between the doctor and the patient/the person consenting on behalf of the patient.

Interpreter's name ....

Interpreter's signature.. **Date:** ....

Witness: .... **Date:**............................

EXAMINATION OF BLOOD STAINS

Physical Examination

Condition of stain:

Description of the source:

Screening Tests

Reaction:

Benzidine/Phenolphthalein test:

Microscopic and Microchemical Tests

Examination for evidence of cells (RBC):

Confirmatory tests:

Principle of the test

a. Hemin crystal test (Teichmann test):

b. Hemochromogen crystal test (Takayama test):

c. Blood grouping:

Opinion

EXAMINATION OF SEMINAL STAINS

Physical Examination

Quantity:

Viscosity:

Odour:

Appearance of the stain:

Chemical Examination

Reaction:

Florence test:

Principle of the test

Barberio test:

Microscopic Examination

Opinion

GUIDELINES FOR CLINICAL EXAMINATION FOR DRUNKENNESS BY GOVERNMENT MEDICAL OFFICER

Objectives

To decide whether:

1. The subject is under the influence of alcohol.
2. His condition is due to illness or injury.
3. It is safe for him to be detained in a police station or he should be admitted to a hospital.

Consent

Obtain informed, written consent.

Preliminary Particulars

Name, age sex, occupation and residential address.

Identification marks: Record at least two permanent marks of identification as for any medicolegal case.

Time of commencement of examination.

Escorts: Record the name and number of escorting police constable, and the police station to which he is attached.

History:

a. Has he consumed alcohol? If so, at what time, and what was the nature and quantity consumed?
b. Is he in the habit of consuming alcohol regularly? If so, since how long and how frequently?
c. Does he suffer from any disease or disability?
d. Is he taking any medication or drug? If so, what is the nature and dose?

Physical Examination

1. *General appearance*: State of clothing, behaviour, disposition, etc.
2. *Speech*: Normal or slurred or overprecise.
3. *Breath*: Odour of alcohol present or absent.
4. *Stance*: Does he sway when standing erect with his feet together and eyes closed?
5. *Gait*: Ask him to walk across the room and observe whether the gait is normal or staggering, straight or irregular. Ask him to stop or turn around and observe whether there is a delay in response (increase reaction time), as well as the manner of turning (whether there is a tendency to fall).
6. *Writing*: Ask him to write or copy a few sentences in the language with which he is familiar. Note the time taken, repitition or omission of words, etc.
7. *Eyes and visual acuity*: Note whether the eyes are reddened, presence or absence of nystagmus, status of pupils, and test for pupillary reaction to light.
8. *Vital data*: Record the pulse, temperature, and blood pressure.
9. *Reflexes*: Normal or depressed.
10. *Muscular coordination*: Test this by asking the individual to perform a new simple tests:
    a. Finger-nose test
    b. Buttoning/unbuttoning shirt
    c. Picking up pencil/pen from the floor

Examination also the cardiovascular, pulmonary, and alimentary systems in the visual way.

Look for the presence of injuries. Pay particular attention to evidence of head injury.

Mental Examination

1. *Memory*: Test for ability to recall recent events. Alternatively, a set of simple data can be told to him at the beginning of the examination, which he is asked to memorize, and at the end of the examination he is asked to recite them.
2. *Orientation*:
   a. To time—Ask him to state the approximate time of day, or the day of the week.
   b. To space—Ask him as to whether he is aware of his present location, the direction in which the entrance to the building lies, etc.

Laboratory Investigations

Collect blood and urine samples. A quick, qualitative urine test for ethanol involves addition of equal volumes of 10% sodium dichromate in 50% H_2SO_4 to the urine sample. Development of green colour indicates the presence of ethanol with reference to the blood sample, about 5 mL drawn from a peripheral vein is usually sufficient. The site to be punctured should not be swabbed with surgical spirit since it can contaminate the blood sample and result in a false positive test for alcohol. Instead the area can be washed with soap and water prior to puncture, and swabbed with spirit after the blood sample has been withdrawn. The collected sample of blood must be preserved in a chemically clean container with sodium fluoride as preservative (50 mg for 5 mL). Some workers believe that it is desirable to add potassium oxalate (15 mg). Refrigeration of the sample or placing it in an icebox is a good alternative. For urine sample, the recommended preservative is phenyl mercuric nitrate. Alternatively, sodium fluoride (50 mg/10 mL) can be used.

Opinion

This should be phrased in **one** of the following ways:

a. The individual examined has not consumed alcohol.
b. The individual examined has consumed alcohol, but is not under its influence.
c. The individual examined has consumed alcohol and is under its influence.

Opinion (a) is given if there is no smell of alcohol in the breath and/or laboratory analysis is negative for alcohol; and all the clinical findings are normal.

Opinion (b) is given if there is smell of alcohol in the breath and/or laboratory analysis reveals the presence of alcohol; but clinical examination reveals only normal findings.

Opinion (c) is given if there is smell of alcohol in the breath and/or laboratory analysis reveals the presence of alcohol; and clinical examination reveals abnormal findings.

Authentication

Signature of the medical officer, his name and designation and the time of concluding the examination.

Toxicology (Study of Poisons)

<table>
<tr><td rowspan="2">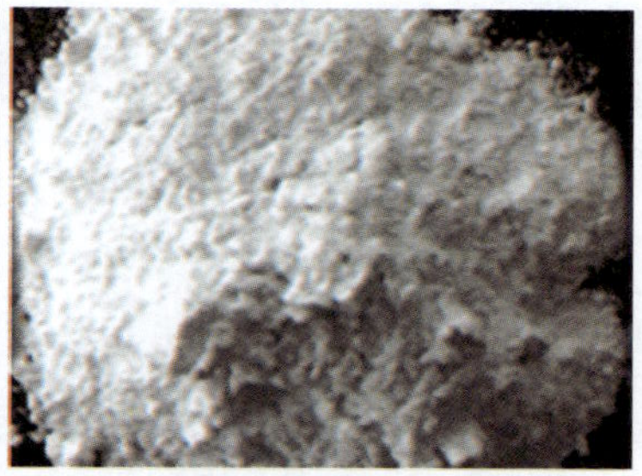
Arsenic trioxide (Amorphous form)</td><td rowspan="2">Description:
White, powder like mass.
Classification: Metallic irritant
Fatal dose (LD 50):
200–300 mg
Fatal period: 12–24 hours</td><td>Clinical features of acute poisoning</td><td>Treatment</td><td>Autopsy finding</td></tr>
<tr><td>A. Fulminant type: Ingestion of massive dose—GI symptoms are absent. Shock and peripheral vascular failure (death occurs with 1–3 hrs)
B. Gastrointestinal type:
1. Severe projectile vomiting.
2. Diarrhea associated with pain abdomen, tenesmus and 'rise water stool'.
CVS: Hypotension, ventricular arrhythmia.
Renal: Oliguria, uremia, hematuria.
Neurological: Asymmetric, distal, 'Gloves-Stocking' distribution of painful peripheral neuropathy</td><td>1. Supportive measures: Gastric lavage, Intravenous fluid, cardiac monitoring.
2. Chelation therapy: This can be done with BAL, DMSA, DMPS or penicillamine.
BAL is started at 3-5 mg/kg deep IM till urinary. As level falls below 50 μg/24 hrs. Usual duration of therapy is 7–10 days.
3. Hemodialysis or exchange transfusion.</td><td>1. Gastrointestinal congestion is prominent. Gastric mucosa may have 'red velvety appearance' due to frank hemorrhagic gastritis. Focal gastric hemorrhages may give rise to 'flea-bitten appearance'.
2. Subendocardial hemorrhages
3. Fatty degeneration of heart, liver, kidney
4. Apart from routine viscera, Arsenic can be detected from long bones, scalp hair and skin.</td></tr>
<tr><td rowspan="2">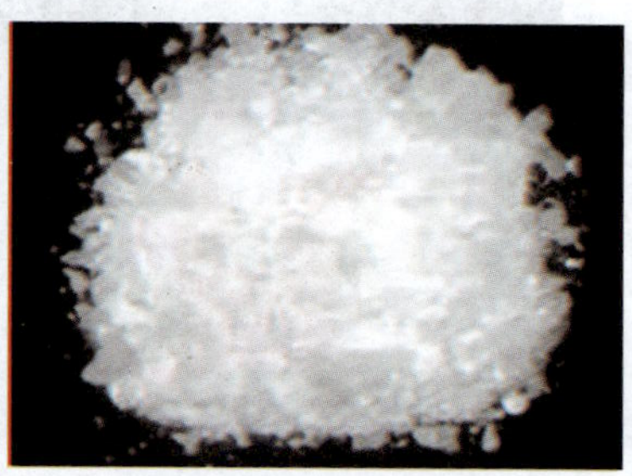</td><td rowspan="2">Description

Classification

Fatal dose (LD50)

Fatal period</td><td>Clinical features</td><td>Treatment</td><td>Autopsy finding</td></tr>
<tr><td></td><td></td><td></td></tr>
</table>

<table>
<tr><td rowspan="2">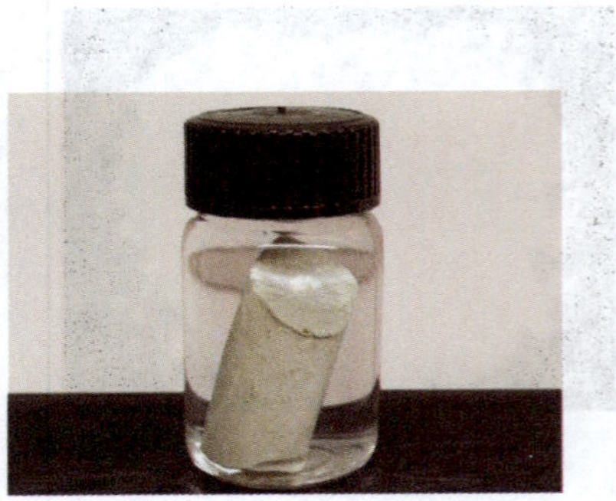</td><td rowspan="2">Description

Classification

Fatal dose (LD50)

Fatal period</td><td>Clinical features</td><td>Treatment</td><td>Autopsy findings</td></tr>
<tr><td></td><td></td><td></td></tr>
<tr><td rowspan="2">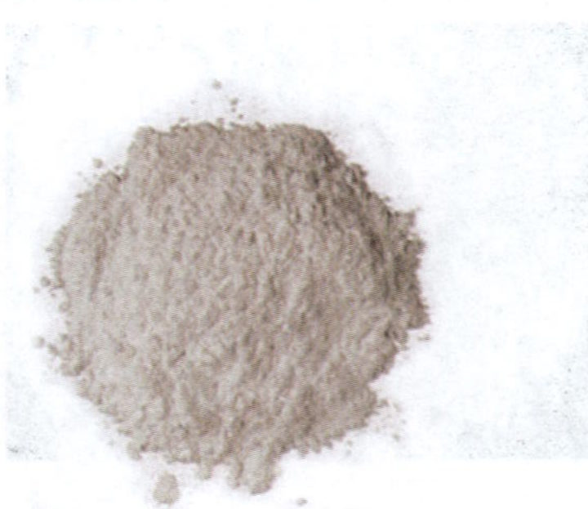</td><td rowspan="2">Description

Classification

Fatal dose (LD50)

Fatal period</td><td>Clinical features</td><td>Treatment</td><td>Autopsy findings</td></tr>
<tr><td></td><td></td><td></td></tr>
</table>

	Description Classification Fatal dose (LD50) Fatal period	*Clinical features*	*Treatment*	*Autopsy findings*
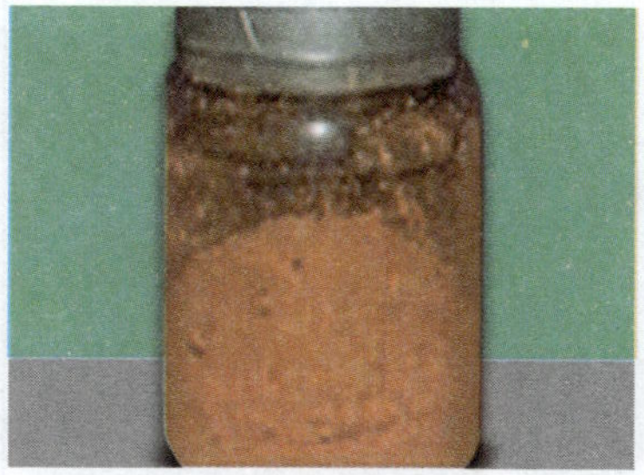	**Description** **Classification** **Fatal dose (LD50)** **Fatal period**			
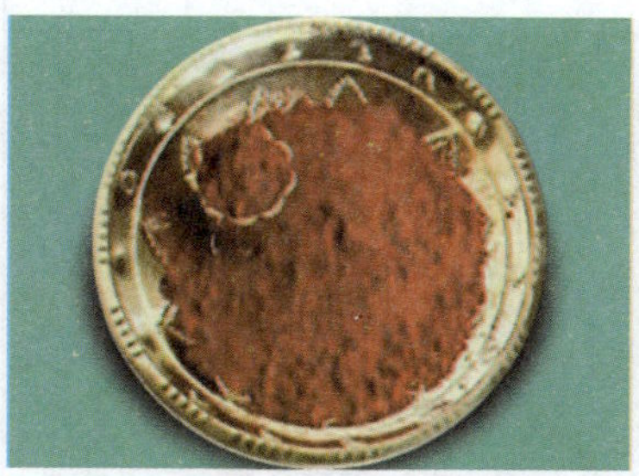	**Description** **Classification** **Fatal dose (LD50)** **Fatal period**	*Clinical features*	*Treatment*	*Autopsy findings*

		Clinical features	*Treatment*	*Autopsy findings*
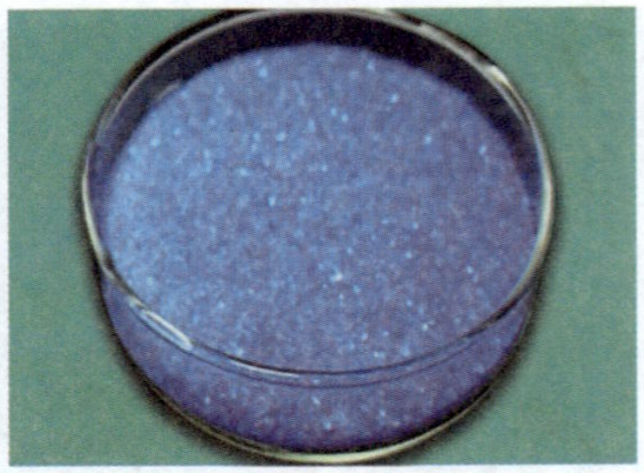	**Description** **Classification** **Fatal dose (LD50)** **Fatal period**			
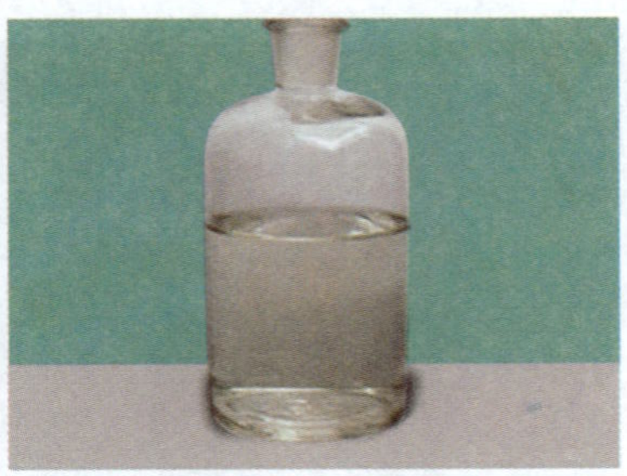	**Description** **Classification** **Fatal dose (LD50)** **Fatal period**	*Clinical features*	*Treatment*	*Autopsy findings*

		Clinical features	*Treatment*	*Autopsy findings*
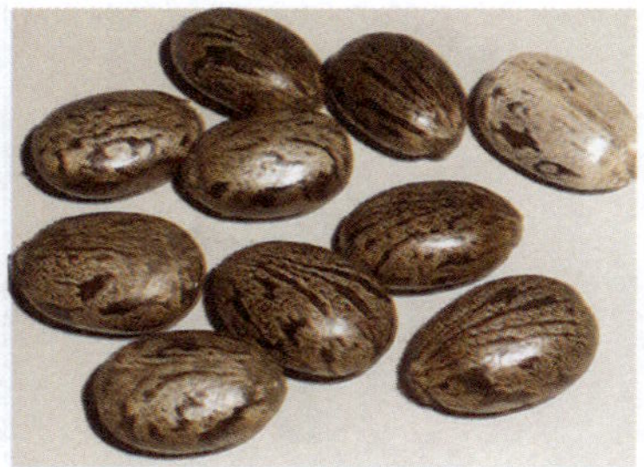	**Description** **Classification** **Fatal dose (LD50)** **Fatal period**			
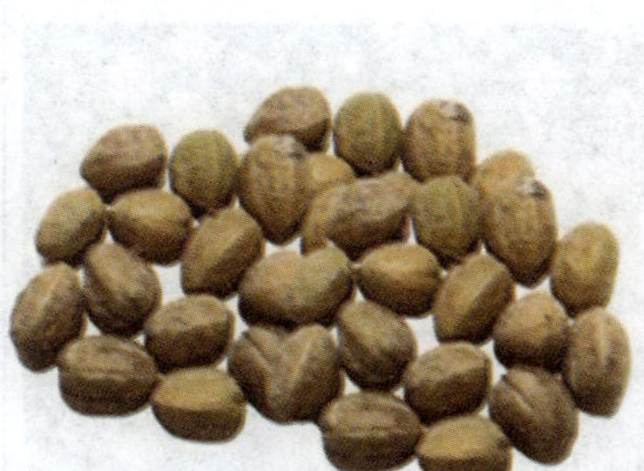	**Description** **Classification** **Fatal dose (LD50)** **Fatal period**	*Clinical features*	*Treatment*	*Autopsy findings*

		Clinical features	Treatment	Autopsy findings
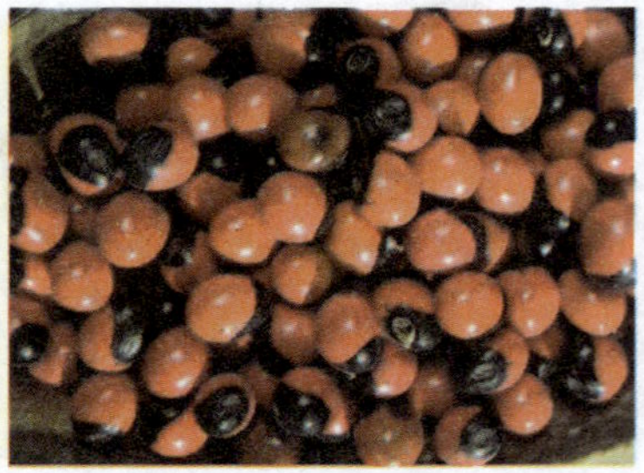	**Description** **Classification** **Fatal dose (LD50)** **Fatal period**			
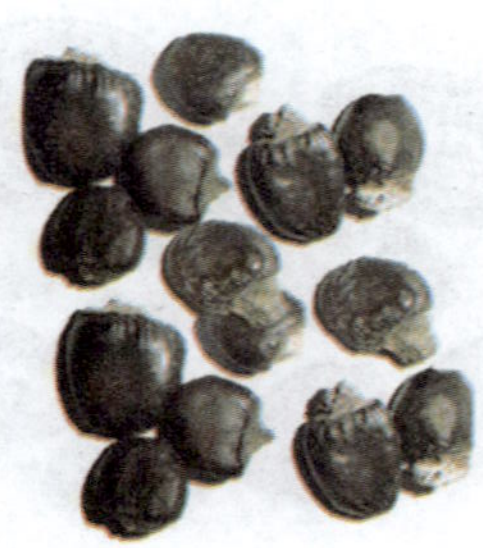	**Description** **Classification** **Fatal dose (LD50)** **Fatal period**			

<table>
<tr><td rowspan="2">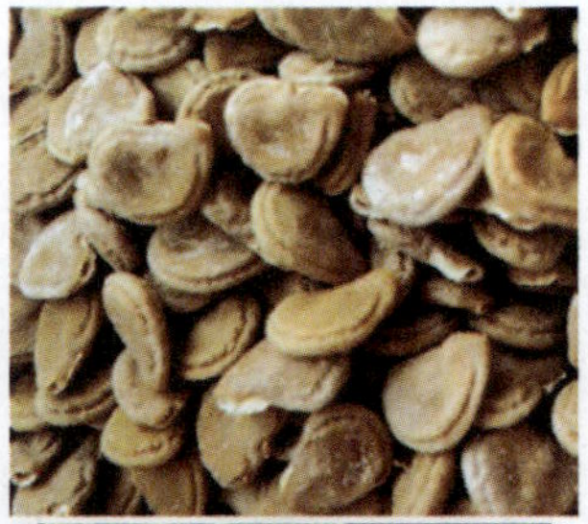
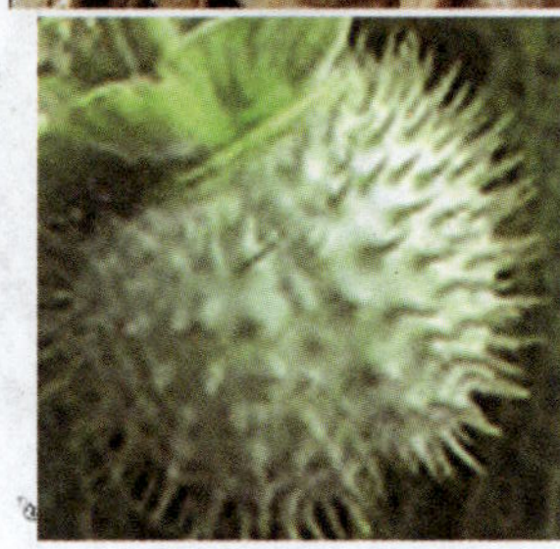</td><td rowspan="2">Description

Classification

Fatal dose (LD50)

Fatal period</td><td>Clinical features</td><td>Treatment</td><td>Autopsy findings</td></tr>
<tr><td></td><td></td><td></td></tr>
<tr><td rowspan="2">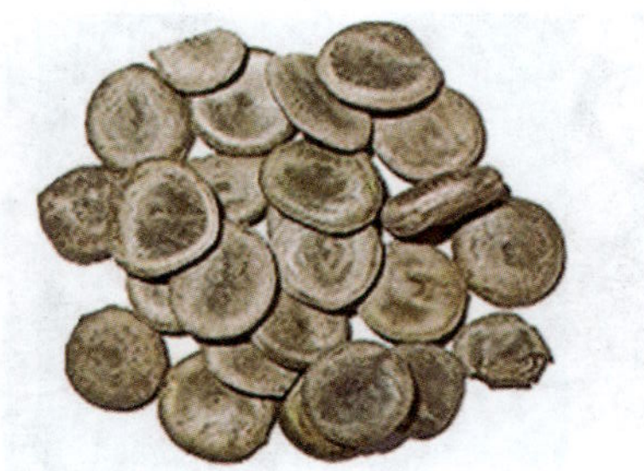</td><td rowspan="2">Description

Classification

Fatal dose (LD50)

Fatal period</td><td>Clinical features</td><td>Treatment</td><td>Autopsy findings</td></tr>
<tr><td></td><td></td><td></td></tr>
</table>

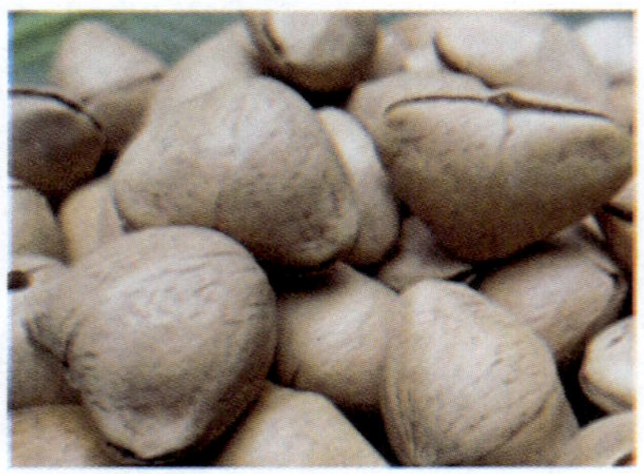	**Description** **Classification** **Fatal dose (LD50)** **Fatal period**	*Clinical features*	*Treatment*	*Autopsy findings*
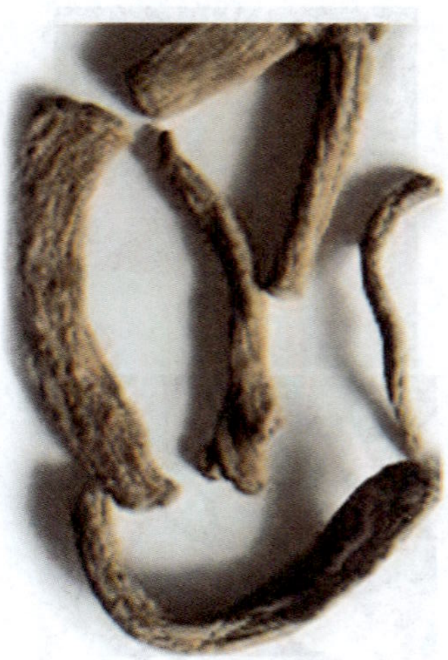	**Description** **Classification** **Fatal dose (LD50)** **Fatal period**	*Clinical features*	*Treatment*	*Autopsy findings*

<table>
<tr><td rowspan="2">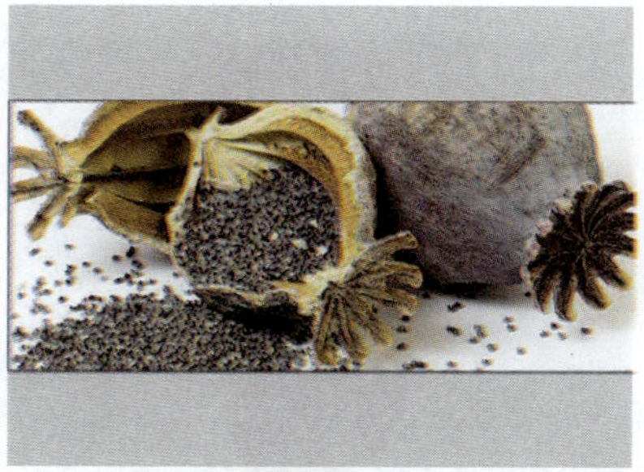</td><td rowspan="2">Description

Classification

Fatal dose (LD50)

Fatal period</td><td>Clinical features</td><td>Treatment</td><td>Autopsy findings</td></tr>
<tr><td></td><td></td><td></td></tr>
<tr><td rowspan="2">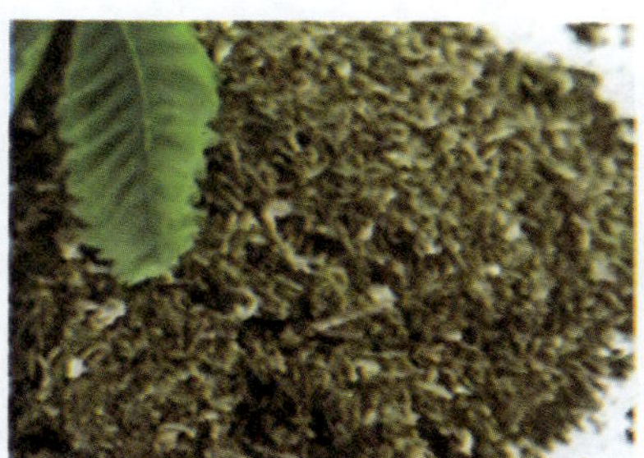</td><td rowspan="2">Description

Classification

Fatal dose (LD50)

Fatal period</td><td>Clinical features</td><td>Treatment</td><td>Autopsy findings</td></tr>
<tr><td></td><td></td><td></td></tr>
</table>

		Clinical features	Treatment	Autopsy findings
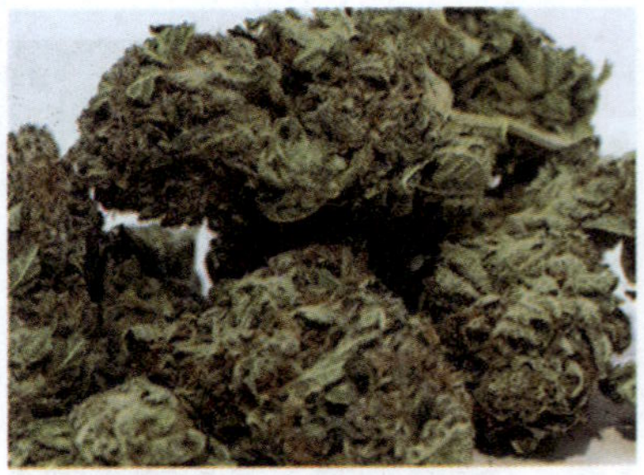	**Description** **Classification** **Fatal dose (LD50)** **Fatal period**			
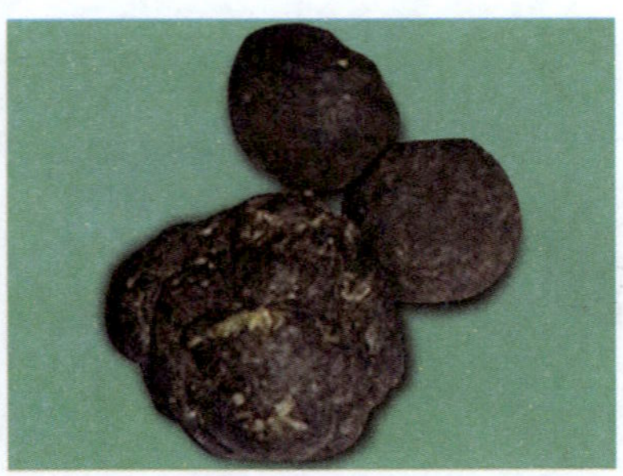	**Description** **Classification** **Fatal dose (LD50)** **Fatal period**			

<table>
<tr><td rowspan="2">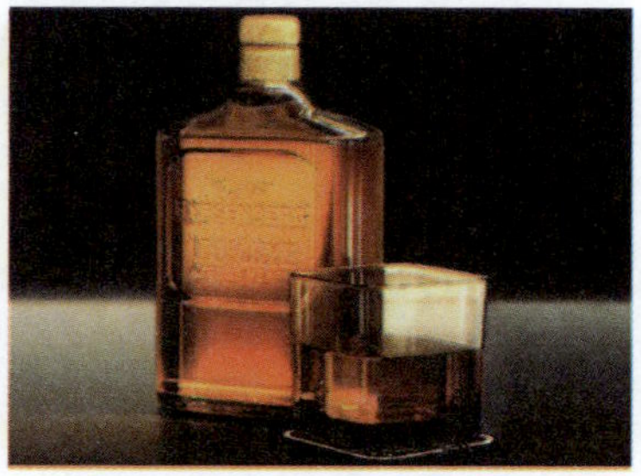</td><td rowspan="2">Description

Classification

Fatal dose (LD50)

Fatal period</td><td>Clinical features</td><td>Treatment</td><td>Autopsy findings</td></tr>
<tr><td></td><td></td><td></td></tr>
<tr><td rowspan="2">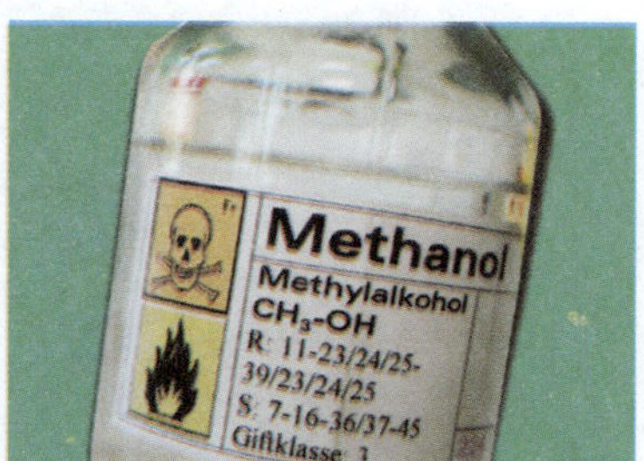</td><td rowspan="2">Description

Classification

Fatal dose (LD50)

Fatal period</td><td>Clinical features</td><td>Treatment</td><td>Autopsy findings</td></tr>
<tr><td></td><td></td><td></td></tr>
</table>

		Clinical features	Treatment	Autopsy findings
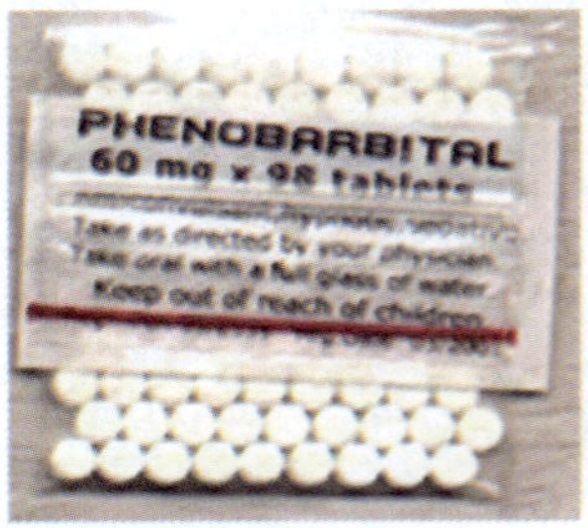	**Description** **Classification** **Fatal dose (LD50)** **Fatal period**			
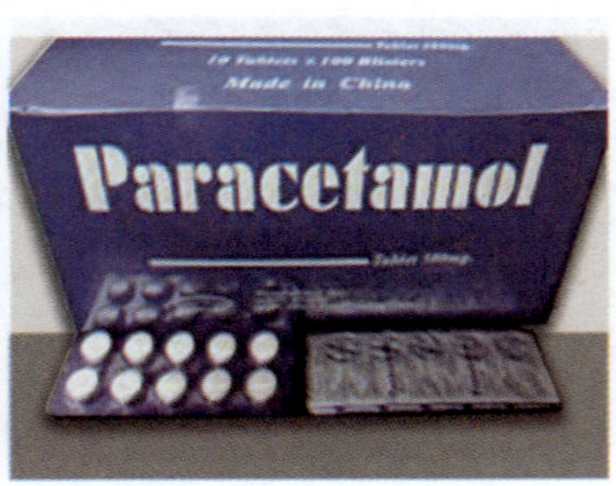	**Description** **Classification** **Fatal dose (LD50)** **Fatal period**			

		Clinical features	Treatment	Autopsy findings
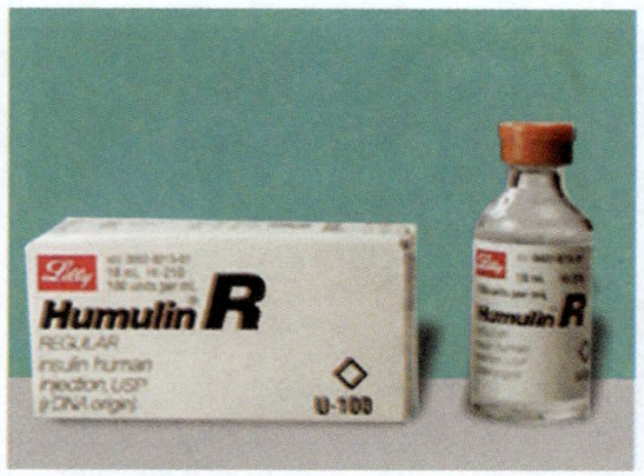	**Description** **Classification** **Fatal dose (LD50)** **Fatal period**			
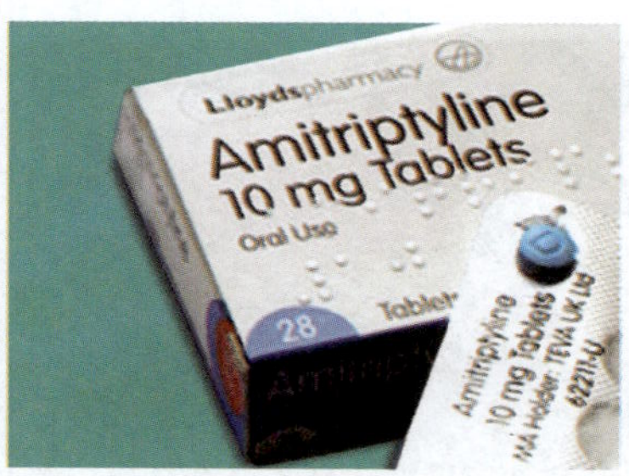	**Description** **Classification** **Fatal dose (LD50)** **Fatal period**			

		Clinical features	Treatment	Autopsy findings
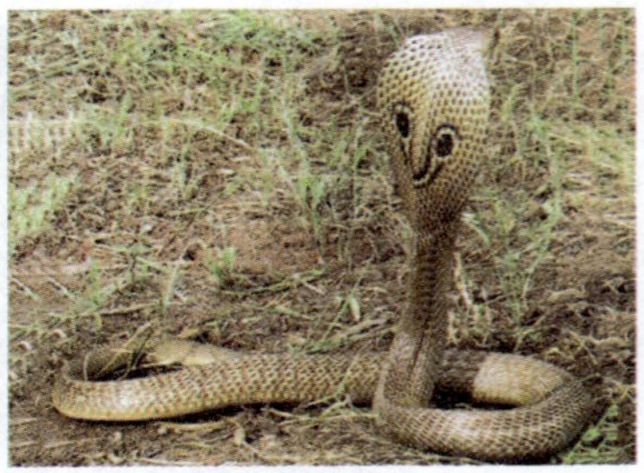	**Description** **Classification** **Fatal dose (LD50)** **Fatal period**			
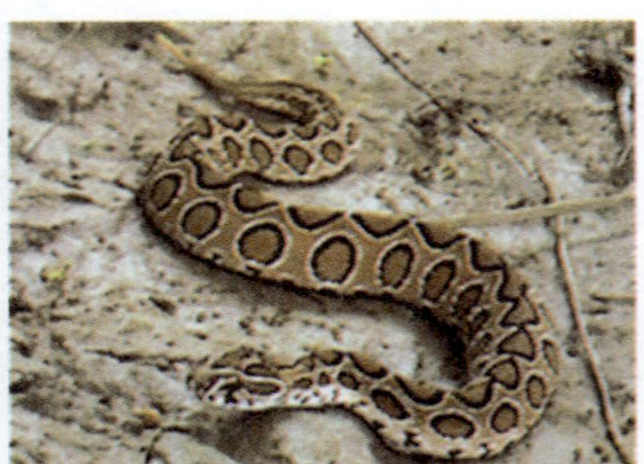	**Description** **Classification** **Fatal dose (LD50)** **Fatal period**			

		Clinical features	Treatment	Autopsy findings
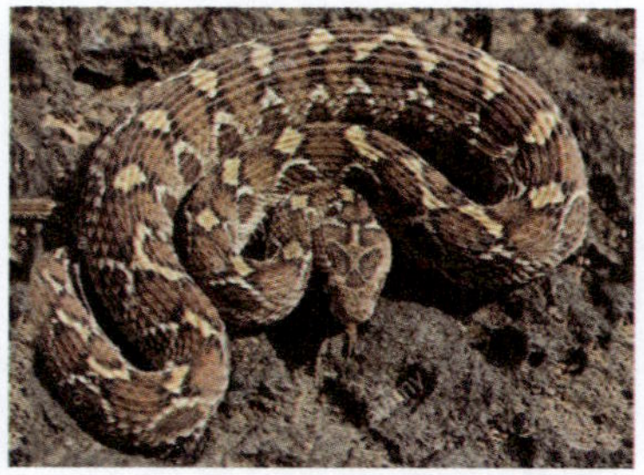	**Description** **Classification** **Fatal dose (LD50)** **Fatal period**			
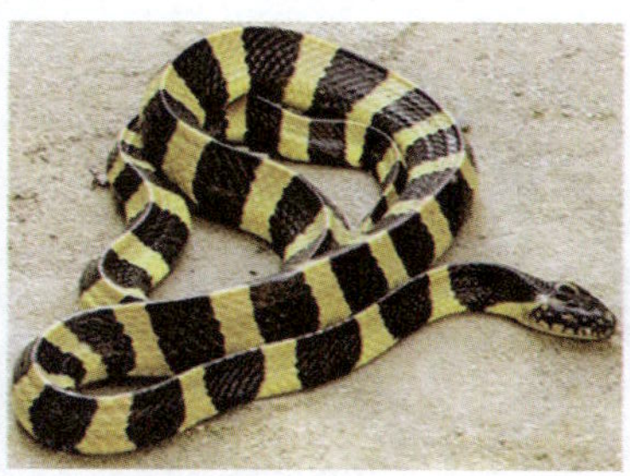	**Description** **Classification** **Fatal dose (LD50)** **Fatal period**			

		Clinical features	*Treatment*	*Autopsy findings*
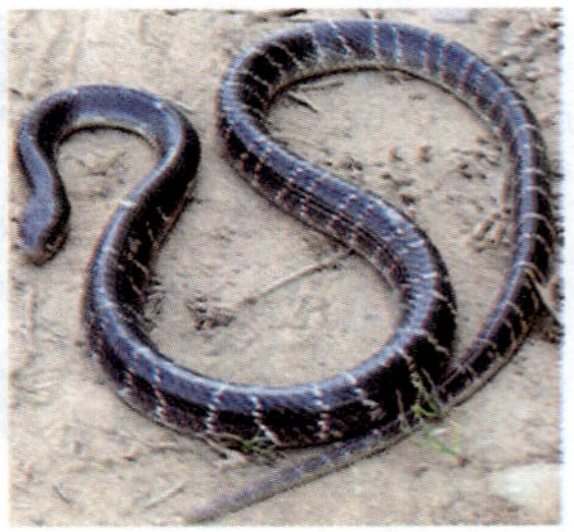	**Description** **Classification** **Fatal dose (LD50)** **Fatal period**			
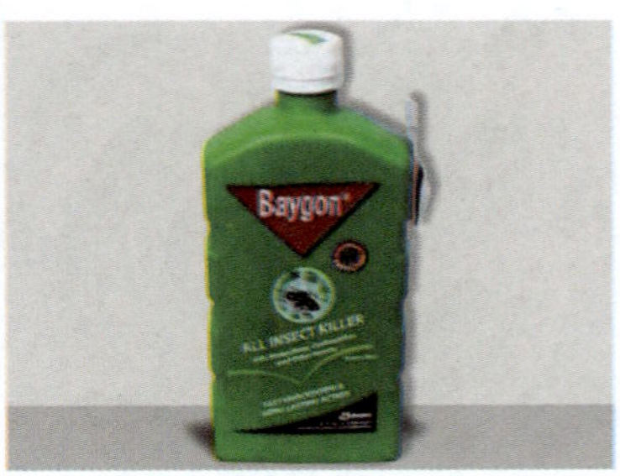 	**Description** **Classification** **Fatal dose (LD50)** **Fatal period**	*Clinical features*	*Treatment*	*Autopsy findings*

MODEL EXERCISE ON PRACTICAL PROBLEMS OF CLINICAL TOXICOLOGY

1. A 35-year-old male was recovered by railway police in disoriented state and brought to ER. Apparently, this guy was a traveller, and he accepted some food from a co-passenger. Thereafter, he became delirious and all his valuables have been robbed. On examination, his skin is dry and red flushed, Temperature = 104° F, pupil bilaterally dilated, he is muttering some incomprehensible words, trying to pick up imaginary things from bed and air.
   a. What is the probable reason for his condition?
   b. What is the active principle?
   c. What is the probable dose in this case?
   d. Name the specific antidote.

....

....

....

....

....

....

....

....

2. A 60-year-old male patient was brought to ER in an unconscious state. On enquiry, it was learnt that he was suffering from end stage hepatocellular carcinoma with multiple metastases, and he was on palliative pain management therapy. On examination, his GCS was 5/15, cyanosis of nailbeds and lips, pupils bilaterally pin pointed and not reacting to light temperature 96° F, SpO_2 = 84%, respiratory rate = 9/min with shallow breathing, peripheries cold, BP = 88/50 mm Hg, A typical heavy musty odour can be appreciated from his mouth.
   a. What is the probable reason for his condition?
   b. What is the specific antidote for this condition?
   c. Name a bedside test for diagnosis.

....

....

....

....

....

....

....

....

3. A 15-year-old boy was brought to ER with C/O burning sensation from mouth to stomach with tingling and numbness, nausea-vomiting, profuse salivation, headache, dizziness, palpitation and feeling of constriction of chest. On enquiry, he gives history of consumption of a root, found in jungle, which he thought as horseradish. O/E, his GCS=15/15, pulse= 180-200/min, grossly irregular and feeble, BP= 70/50 mmHg. While testing pupillary light reaction, pupils seen to contract and dilate alternately. His ECG strip is given below:

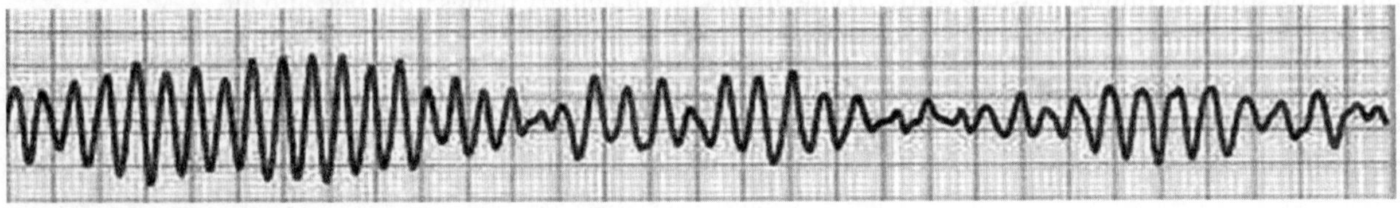

   a. What is the probable diagnosis for this condition?
   b. What is the active principle?
   c. What is the mechanism of action?
   d. Is it an ideal homicidal poison? Give reasons.

4. A 14-year-old girl was brought to ER with C/O recurrent convulsions for last 2 hours. On enquiry, the girl gives history of consumption of some button like seeds. The convulsions are lasting for 2–3 minutes and in between two successive convulsive episodes, the muscles are completely relaxed.
   a. What is the name of the seeds that the girl had consumed?
   b. What is the active principle?
   c. What is the mechanism of action of it?
   d. Which is the name of the infective disease that closely resembles this condition, and how will you differentiate between these two?

5. On the day of Diwali, a man invites his unmarried uncle, who is creating much problems with his property, to his house and offers whisky. The uncle, who is an occasional drinker, finds the whisky more bitter than usual. After having the drink, the person feels a little restless. Then he experiences muscle stiffness and twitching, which soon turns into convulsive movements. Relatives rushed him to the hospital. On the way to hospital, the body bends backwards like an arch, angles of mouth is drawn back. In between two paroxysms of convulsions, the patient's muscle are completely relaxed.
   a. What is the poison responsible for the situation?
   b. What is the mechanism of action of the poison?
   c. Name the active principle.
   d. What is the possible differential diagnosis and how to differentiate between them?

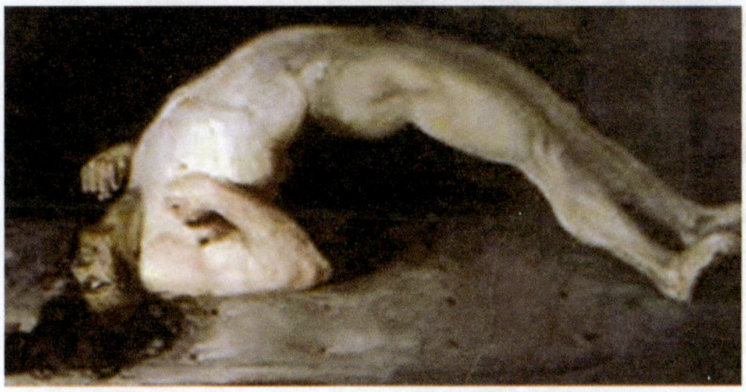

....

....

....

....

....

....

....

....

....

....

....

....

....

....

6. Rahimpur is a small underprivileged village in southern Bengal. The sole water supply for the villagers are deep tubewells and deep wells, which are rarely reformed. Dr Das, the medical officer in local PHC, has noticed a high incidence dermatological disorders among the inhabitants. Most of them present with multiple hard wart-like growth on palm and soles, finely mottled brown pigmentation, irregularly thick and brittle nails, dry fuzzy hair which easily falls off. Many of them also suffer from various skin cancers.

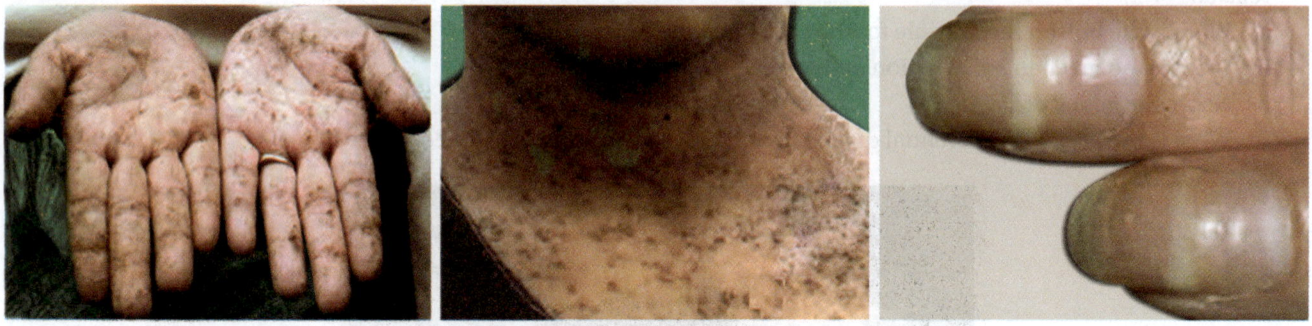

   a. What is the agent responsible for such outbreak?
   b. How will you confirm the diagnosis?
   c. Outline the treatment of this condition.

7. A 30-year-old woodcutter was brought to the ER by this coworkers. He gives a history of being bitten by a snake. His coworkers had killed that snake and brought it along with. The dead snake was about 4 feet in length with triangular head, narrow neck, head covered by small scales, pupil vertical, short tapering tail. On examination, the victim had two pinpoint punctured marks over right ankle, with blood and fluid oozing out from the wound, surrounded by spreading haemorrhagic and necrosed zone. In spite of adequate therapy, the victim succumbed after 12 hours.

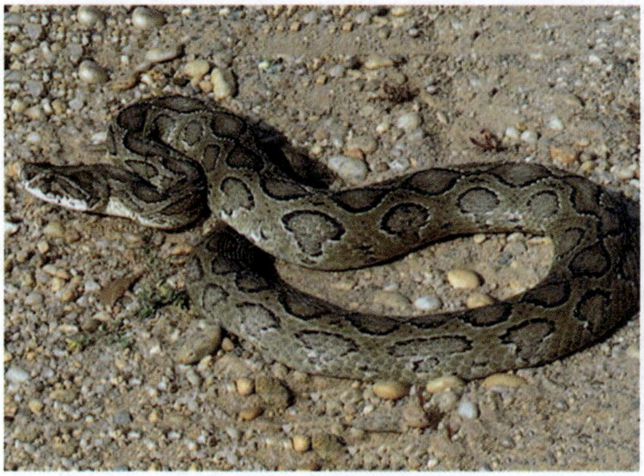

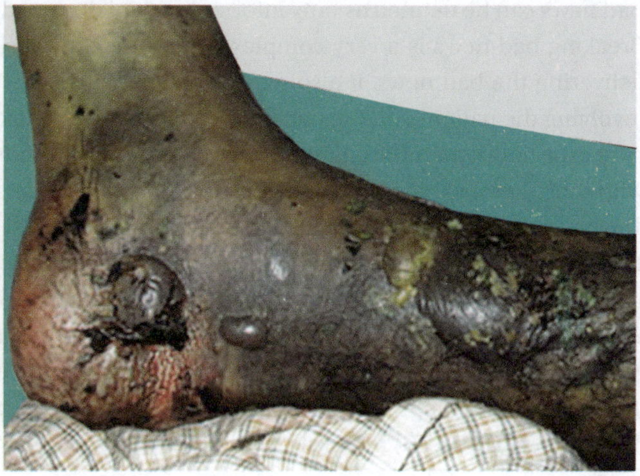

   a. What is the probable cause of death?
   b. Which type of snake was culprit in this case?
   c. What important findings do you expect during autopsy?

PRACTICE ON DEVELOPMENT OF AFFECTIVE SKILLS

Breaking of Bad News

SPIKES—A Six-Step Protocol for Delivering Bad News:

Bad news can be defined as "any information which can adversely affect an individual's view of his or her future.

Breaking bad news is a very complex communication task. In addition to the verbal communication skill of actually delivering the bad news, it also requires other skills. These are responding properly to patients' emotional reactions, involving the patient and the patient party in decision-making, handling the stress created by patients' expectations for cure especially when the chance of cure is extremely remote, the involvement of multiple family members and dealing with their various issues and demands related to the treatment.

The basic goal is to help the clinician to meet the four most important objectives of the interview disclosing bad news:

1. To collect information from the patient and patient party to allow the physician to understand the patient's knowledge and specially expectations and readiness to hear the bad news
2. To transmit the medical information to them accordingly to the patient's needs and desires
3. To provide mental support to the patient to reduce the emotional impact.
4. To seek the patient's cooperation in developing a strategy for treatment plan for the future.

The protocol **(SPIKES)** has of six steps.

STEP 1: S—SETTING UP the Interview:

....

The following guidelines may help the clinician to achieve this step satisfactorily:

- ***Arrange for some privacy*** in form of a separate interview room, if possible, but, if one is not available, the clinician can put curtains around the patient's bed.
- ***Involve significant other family members*** because most of the patients want to have someone else with them. In such a case, the clinician can ask the patient to choose one or two family representatives.
- ***Sit down*** and ask the patient and his family members to sit so that the patient should realize that you will not rush.
- ***Make proper connection with the patient*** like maintaining eye contact which is an important way of establishing rapport, touching the patient on the arm or holding a hand (if the patient is comfortable with this) is another way to achieve this.
- ***Manage time constraints and interruptions:*** Inform the patient and his family members of any time constraints, you may have or he or she has. Set your mobile on silent mode to avoid interruptions and distractions.

STEP 2: P—Assessing the Patient's PERCEPTION

Before directly going to the medical findings, the clinician should use open-ended questions to create a reasonably accurate picture of how the patient perceives the current medical situation

For example, the clinician should ask, "What have you been told about your medical situation or diagnosis so far?" or "What do you think the reasons we did the MRI/CT scan/Chest X-ray?". Based on this information, the clinician can correct any misinformation, and trailor the bad news accordingly to realize what the patient understands.

STEP 3: I—Obtaining the Patient's INVITATION

Clinicians should keep it in mind that while a majority of patients express their desire for full information about their diagnosis, prognosis, and details of their illness, some patients do not. Now when a clinician hears a patient expresses explicitly his or her wish for complete information, it may lessen the anxiety associated with divulging the bad news. However, avoiding deliberately information is a valid psychological coping mechanism and may be more likely to be manifested later as the illness becomes more severe.

Examples of questions the clinician can ask the patient would be:

"How would you like me to give the information about the test results?

Would you like me to give you all the information or sketch out the results and spend more time discussing the treatment plan?".

If patients do not want to know details, offer to answer any questions, they may have in the future or to talk to a relative or friend in that situation with proper documentation in BHT/outdoor ticket.

STEP 4: K—Giving KNOWLEDGE and Information to the Patient

Prior warning the patient that bad news is coming may lessen the mental shock that can occur following the disclosure of bad news and may facilitate the clinician during information processing. Examples of phrases that can be used like:

"Unfortunately I've got some bad news to tell you" or "I'm sorry to tell you that..."

Giving medical facts, the one-way part of the physician-patient dialogue, may be improved by a few simple guidelines:

First, assess the level of comprehension and vocabulary of the patient by asking his educational qualification, profession, etc.

Second, try to avoid medical terms and use nontechnical words such as "spread" instead of "metastasized" and "sample of tissue" instead of "biopsy."

Third, avoid excessive bluntness (e.g. "You have very bad cancer and unless you get treatment immediately, you are going to die or there is no cure of the bad cancer you have been diagnosed.") as it is likely to leave the patient isolated and later angry, with a tendency to blame the messenger of the bad news.

Fourth, give information in small chunks and check periodically whether the patient understood it at all.

Fifth, when the prognosis is poor, avoid using phrases such as "There is nothing more we can do for you." This attitude is inconsistent with the fact that patients often have other important therapeutic goals such as good pain control and symptomatic relief.

STEP 5: E—Addressing the Patient's EMOTIONS with Empathic Responses

Responding to the patient's emotions is the most difficult challenge of breaking bad news. Patients' emotional reactions may vary from denial, anger, silence to disbelief, crying.

When patient gets the bad news his or her emotional reaction is often an expression of shock and grief. In this situation, the physician should offer support to the patient by making an empathic response. An empathic response consists of four steps:

- First, observe for any emotion on the part of the patient after getting the bad news. This may be tearfulness, a look of sadness, silence.
- Second, If a patient appears sad but is silent, use open questions to query the patient as to what they are thinking or feeling.
- Third, identify the reason for the emotion. This is usually connected to the bad news. However, if you are not sure, again, ask the patient.
- Fourth, after you have allowed the patient a brief period of time to express his or her feelings, let the patient know that you have connected the emotion with the reason for the emotion by making a connecting statement. An example:
  - ***Doctor:*** I am sorry to say that the X-ray shows that the chemotherapy does not seem to be working [pause]. Unfortunately, the tumour has grown somewhat beyond the capacity of chemotherapy [pause].
  - ***Patient:*** I have been afraid of the same doctor! [Cries]

- ***Doctor:*** [Moves his chair closer, offers the patient a tissue, and pauses.] I know that this is not what you wanted to hear. I wish the news were better....[pause]

In the above dialogue, the physician observed the patient was crying and realized that the patient was tearful because of the bad news. He moved closer to the patient. At this point, he might have also touched the patient's arm or hand, if they were both comfortable and paused a moment to allow him or her to get the composure.

Until an emotion is cleared, it will be extremely difficult on the part of the clinician to go on to discuss other issues. If the emotion does not diminish shortly, it is beneficial to continue to make empathic responses until the patient becomes calm. Clinicians can also use empathic responses to acknowledge their own sadness like "I also wish the news were better". It can be a show of support to follow the empathic response with a validating statement, which lets the patient know that their feelings are legitimate.

STEP 6: S—STRATEGY and SUMMARY

- Plan the discussion in advance
- Create a comfortable setting
- Encourage family/friend presence
- Assess patient's ability to discuss bad news
- Confirm patient's understanding of cancer
- Assess how much patient wants to know
- Organize a strategy for disclosing information
- Include family/caregiver in discussion
- Provide information in small increments
- Avoid medical jargon
- Check to see, if information was correctly received by patient
- Reinforce and clarify information
- Detect anxiety
- Detect sadness
- Handle the patient's emotional reactions
- Respond empathetically.

Task

1. **Mr Shyamal Roy, a 56-year-old mechanical engineer is a chronic smoker for last 20 years. He along with his wife came to your chamber with the CT scan chest report which you had advised on his last visit. CT scan revealed CA Lungs with axillary lymph node metastasis. Now you have to break the bad news to him and his wife.**
2. **Subham, a 20-year-old male subject was admitted under you in Intensive Trauma Care unit with history of bike accident. He was put on a ventilator. In spite of all available treatment modalities Subham died after 1 day of hospital admission. Being in the position of ITU in-charge, you have to give the bad news to his family members.**

Informed Consent Interview

Problem: Kamal, a 21-year-old male accused under Sec 376 IPC, was brought to the Department of Forensic Medicine and Toxicology by SI Ranjit Mukherjee of Entally PS for medicolegal examination vide Entally PS Case No 235 dated 14/10/17 under 376 IPC. Take an informed consent for medicolegal examination.

Guidelines

Points to be checked by the evaluator	*Whether done by the examinee (put tick or cross)*
1. Asked the accompanying police person to remove the ropes tied around waist and hands	
2. Asked the police person to wait outside the examination room	
3. Asked for the disinterested third party to be present during taking the informed consent	
4. Greeted the subject	
5. Asked the subject to sit	
6. Asked the preferred language for communication	
7. Self introduction	
8. Created a rapport with the subject	
9. Assessed the compos mentis of the subject to check whether he could give a legally valid consent	
10. Discussed the purpose of the examination	
11. Discussed the possible outcome of the examination	
12. Disclosed that the report will be supplied to the concerned authority and the same may be produced in Court in future	
13. Revealed that identification marks would be noted with the explanation of its importance	
14. Revealed that photographs if required will be taken for evidential purpose and the same will be supplied to the concerned authority	
15. Revealed that the subject had to undress fully during examination	
16. Discussed in details the steps of physical examination including examination of external genitalia, dental examination and radiological examination, if necessary	
17. Informed in details regarding collection of specimens during examination and the collected specimen will be forwarded to the concerned authority	
18. Revealed that he may be referred to other speciality, if needed	
19. Given chance to the subject any question and any concern of the subject and clarified the queries accordingly and satisfactorily	
20. Informed the subject about his rights of informed refusal before or any time during examination and possible consequences of such refusal	

PROBLEMS ON MEDICAL NEGLIGENCE

Dr A performed an appendicectomy operation on Ms X. On discharge, the patient was stable except with some amount of pain at the operating site. Her pain increased with time. On 5th day after discharge, she also developed fever. Her house physician advised a repeat USG of whole abdomen. In the report, the radiologist noted a metallic object at the right iliac fossa. Three days later Ms X underwent another laparotomy operation and a mosquito forceps was recovered from the operating field of the previous operation. The patient filed a negligence suite against Dr A.

Do you consider the negligence suite is rational? Justify your answer with reasoning.

(Guideline: Write considering the following points: Observation, Discussion, Reasoning, Opinion)

WET SPECIMEN

AUTOPSY
AUTOPSY CASE (10)
EXAMINATION OF SKELETAL REMAINS

Requisition from ....Case No. of PS .... Date...
Brought by .... PC No. .... PS ....
Description

(**Guideline**: Whether the bones are human or not?
If human, whether they are male or female?
Whether they belong to one or more individuals?
The stature of the individual to whom the bones belonged.
The age of the individual to whom the bones belonged.
The time since death.
Whether the bones have been cut, sawn, gnawed by animals or burnt?
The probable cause of death.)

Opinion: (Answer to the question as mentioned in the guideline)

(Signature of MO with seal)

The bundle of bones, packed and sealed, handed over to PC.................................. No......... PS............................ along with the sample seal.

(Signature of Police Constable (PC))

MODEL PRACTICAL QUESTION PAPER
Forensic Medicine and Toxicology (PRACTICAL)

Time: 40 minutes **Full Marks: 40**

There are four groups of questions each carrying 08 marks

(Time: Spotting 2 min each, Exercise: 8 min each. Total: 40 min)

1. Spotting **8**
   i. Identify the tooth marked 'A'. Write its age of eruption. What is the total number of teeth in the oral cavity at this age? **1 + ½ + ½ = 2**
   ii. Identify the first carpal bone to appear in the given skiagram. Determine whether the individual is an adult or not with one point in favour of your opinion. **1 + ½ + ½ = 2**
   iii. Identify the poison that causes constriction of the pupil. Write its antidote and route of administration. **1 + ½ + ½ = 2**
   iv. Identify the photography showing the intracranial haemorrhage in which lucid interval is common. Name the commonest site and source of bleeding in such type of intracranial haemorrhage. **1 + ½ + ½ = 2**
2. Draft a Medical certificate of cause of death from the given data. **8**
   Mr X a 65-year-old hypertensive and diabetic male was admitted to the hospital in ICU last night with history of chest pain, respiratory distress and palpitation. On examination, there was hypotension and tachycardia. Echocardiographic examination revealed cardiac tamponade with rupture of right ventricle. He had a past history of myocardial infarction 6 months ago. The patient died this morning at 5.30 AM.
3. Prepare an injury report from the given data (***with a projection/model/photograph***) **8**
   Name: XYZ, Age - 30 yrs, Sex - Male. ID marks—Mole on right side face, scar over left eyebrow. Brought by—C/251 XY of ABC PS.
   History of physical assault by wooden stick.
   Injuries:
   1. Abrasion on the right forearm.
   2. Bruise on left scapular region.
   3. Lacerated wound on right parietal region of head.
4. The following ligature materials were recovered from the scene of crime (nylon rope/electric wire/dupatta). From the given photograph of the deceased determine which may be the possible ligature material used. Write the internal findings in the neck of such a case **(Similar questions can be structured using Bones and X-rays, Photograph and Weapons, Autopsy-related materials or Mannequins or Plasticine models).** **8**
5. A 40-year-old male patient presented with a history of pain abdomen, constipation, features of encephalopathy and foot drop. Identify the poison from the supplied specimens given which may have caused the toxicity. Write the blood picture of such a case and the antidote used in the management. **8**

ANNEXURE

LIST OF VISCERA TO BE PRESERVED IN SUSPECTED CASE OF POISONING (FOR CHEMICAL ANALYSIS OF POISON)

- Stomach and whole of its contents.
- The upper part of small intestine with its contents, about 30 cm (Whole intestine in infant).
- A portion of liver (At least 500 g for adults, whole of liver in case of infants).
- Longitudinal half of each kidney.

Hollow viscera (Stomach, Intestine) and solid viscera (Liver, Kidney) should ideally be preserved in separate containers with preservative.

PRESERVATIVES FOR CHEMICAL ANALYSIS OF POISON

- Saturated solution of common salt (SS of NaCl)—Most commonly used
- Alcohol and rectified spirit (Ideal preservative)—contraindications: Carbolic acid, paraldehyde, phosphorous, alcohol, acetic acid, etc.
- Blood: Thymol
- Urine: Thymol

**FORMALIN IS NEVER USED AS PRESERVATIVE FOR THIS PURPOSE

UNDER SPECIAL CIRCUMSTANCES

- Brain—in suspected barbiturate, strychnine, cyanide, OP compounds, anaesthetics and volatile poisoning.
- Spinal cord (entire length)—in strychnine, gelsemium
- Heart—in strychnine, digitalis, yellow oleander.
- Skin—in suspected deaths due to hypodermic injections of substances such as insulin, morphine, cocaine or in corrosive poisoning.
- Nails, hair, bone—in heavy metal poisoning (Inorganic, metallic, irritant poisoning)
- Blood:
  - Generally 100 mg sodium fluoride and 30 mg potassium oxalate for 10 mL of blood as preservative
  - Preserved with sodium citrate in oxalic acid, ethylene glycol, fluoride, CO poisoning.
  - In case of cocaine, plastic bottle should be avoided
  - In case of volatile poisons, a thin layer of liquid paraffin is put over the top of blood column.
- Lung—Gaseous poison, anaesthetic agents, HCN, alcohol, etc.
- Uterus—in criminal abortion and pregnancy
- Finger tips: Unidentified body (preserved in Formalin)
- Urine: 100 mg Sodium Fluoride or 100 mg thymol for 10 mL of urine as preservative. Toluene is better.

NB:

1. The quantity of preservative should be equal or more than that of viscera.
2. Only 2/3rd capacity of bottle to be filled with viscera with preservatives.
3. Bottles should be properly packed, sealed, labelled (as below). If contains infectious or radioactive material, a clearly visible warning to be put on the label.

- In case of volatile poisons or anaesthetic agents, viscera are kept inside an impermeable nylon bag and air-tight packing to avoid evaporation of the poisons.
- A sample of the preservative used, is kept separately and sent along with viscera as control.
- ** All the preserved materials must be properly sealed and labelled before handing over to the authorized police. Police must give receipt for all the materials under his signature and designation.

SAMPLE OF LABEL

.... Police Morgue

PM No .... Date ....

Ref: ....

Name ....

Age .... Sex .... Religion ....

Viscera: Stomach and whole of its content, 500 g of Liver, Lateral surface of each kidney

Urine/Blood: With/Without any preservative

Sample of Preservative: Saturated solution of NaCl/Rectified Spirit

Signature of Autopsy Surgeon

West Bengal Form No. 5372

POSTMORTEM REPORT

(P.R.B. Form No. 55 - Vide Rule 284)

STATION ....

...............day of...........20.....

	Name, sex, age and caste	Whence brought: Village and Thana	Name of Constable by whom brought and names of relatives accompanying	Date and hour of Despatch	Date and hour of Arrival at dead-house	Date and hour of Examination	Information furnished by Police	By whom identified before the Medical Officer

N. B. - Observe the state of all the organs and when no disease or inury is found write "Healthy"

I. EXTERNAL APPEARANCE	1. Condition of subject—stout, emaciated, decomposed etc.	2. Wounds—position, size, character	3. Bruises—position, size and nature	4. Marks of ligature on neck, dissection etc.

II. CRANIUM AND SPINAL CANAL	1. Scalp: Skull and vertebrae	2. Membrane	3. Brain and spinal cord (The spinal canal need not be examined unless any indication of disease or injury exists)

III. THORAX	1. Walls, ribs and cartilages	2. Pleurae	3. Larynx and trachea	Right lung	Left lung	Pericardium	Heart	Vessels

IV. ABDOMEN	1. Walls	2. Peritoneum	3. Mouth, pharynx and esophagus	4. Stomach and its contents	5. Small intestine and its contents	6. Large intestine and its contents

IV. ABDOMEN	7. Liver	8. Spleen	9. Kidneys	10. Bladder	11. Organs of generation, external and internal

MUSCLES, BONES AND JOINTS	1. Injury	2. Disease or deformity	3. Fracture	4. Dislocation

MORE DETAILED DESCRIPTION OF INJURY OR DISEASE	

OPINION OF THE MEDICAL OFFICER AS TO THE CAUSE OF DEATH	REMARKS BY CIVIL SURGEON
N.B. In the case of wounded note whether there is any indication of the wounds being homicidal, sucidal or otherwise *Assistant Surgeon of*..	*Civil Surgeon of*.. *The* *day of* *20*

West Bengal Form No. 5372

POSTMORTEM REPORT

(P.R.B. Form No. 55 - Vide Rule 284)

STATION ....

...............day of...........20.....

	Name, sex, age and caste	Whence brought: Village and Thana	Name of Constable by whom brought and names of relatives accompanying	Date and hour of			Information furnished by Police	By whom identified before the Medical Officer
				Despatch	Arrival at dead-house	Examination		

N. B. - Observe the state of all the organs and when no disease or inury is found write "Healthy"

I. EXTERNAL APPEARANCE	1. Condition of subject—stout, emaciated, decomposed etc.	2. Wounds—position, size, character	3. Bruises—position, size and nature	4. Marks of ligature on neck, dissection etc.

II. CRANIUM AND SPINAL CANAL	1. Scalp: Skull and vertebrae	2. Membrane	3. Brain and spinal cord (The spinal canal need not be examined unless any indication of disease or injury exists)

III. THORAX	1. Walls, ribs and cartilages	2. Pleurae	3. Larynx and trachea	Right lung	Left lung	Pericardium	Heart	Vessels

IV. ABDOMEN	1. Walls	2. Peritoneum	3. Mouth, pharynx and esophagus	4. Stomach and its contents	5. Small intestine and its contents	6. Large intestine and its contents
	7. Liver	8. Spleen	9. Kidneys	10. Bladder	11. Organs of generation, external and internal	

MUSCLES, BONES AND JOINTS	1. Injury	2. Disease or deformity	3. Fracture	4. Dislocation

MORE DETAILED DESCRIPTION OF INJURY OR DISEASE	

OPINION OF THE MEDICAL OFFICER AS TO THE CAUSE OF DEATH	REMARKS BY CIVIL SURGEON
N.B. In the case of wounded note whether there is any indication of the wounds being homicidal, sucidal or otherwise *Assistant Surgeon of...*	*Civil Surgeon of..* *The day of 20*

West Bengal Form No. 5372

POSTMORTEM REPORT

(P.R.B. Form No. 55 - Vide Rule 284)

STATION ....

..............day of..........20.....

	Name, sex, age and caste	Whence brought: Village and Thana	Name of Constable by whom brought and names of relatives accompanying	Date and hour of			Information furnished by Police	By whom identified before the Medical Officer
				Despatch	Arrival at dead-house	Examination		

N. B. - Observe the state of all the organs and when no disease or inury is found write "Healthy"

I. EXTERNAL APPEARANCE	1. Condition of subject—stout, emaciated, decomposed etc.	2. Wounds—position, size, character	3. Bruises—position, size and nature	4. Marks of ligature on neck, dissection etc.

II. CRANIUM AND SPINAL CANAL	1. Scalp: Skull and vertebrae	2. Membrane	3. Brain and spinal cord (The spinal canal need not be examined unless any indication of disease or injury exists)

III. THORAX	1. Walls, ribs and cartilages	2. Pleurae	3. Larynx and trachea	Right lung	Left lung	Pericardium	Heart	Vessels

IV. ABDOMEN	1. Walls	2. Peritoneum	3. Mouth, pharynx and esophagus	4. Stomach and its contents	5. Small intestine and its contents	6. Large intestine and its contents
	7. Liver	8. Spleen	9. Kidneys	10. Bladder	11. Organs of generation, external and internal	

MUSCLES, BONES AND JOINTS	1. Injury	2. Disease or deformity	3. Fracture	4. Dislocation

MORE DETAILED DESCRIPTION OF INJURY OR DISEASE	

OPINION OF THE MEDICAL OFFICER AS TO THE CAUSE OF DEATH	REMARKS BY CIVIL SURGEON
N.B. In the case of wounded note whether there is any indication of the wounds being homicidal, sucidal or otherwise *Assistant Surgeon of.......................*	*Civil Surgeon of.......................* *The day of 20*

West Bengal Form No. 5372

POSTMORTEM REPORT

(P.R.B. Form No. 55 - Vide Rule 284)

STATION ....

...............day of...........20.....

	Name, sex, age and caste	Whence brought: Village and Thana	Name of Constable by whom brought and names of relatives accompanying	Date and hour of			Information furnished by Police	By whom identified before the Medical Officer
				Despatch	Arrival at dead-house	Examination		

N. B. - Observe the state of all the organs and when no disease or inury is found write "Healthy"

I. EXTERNAL APPEARANCE	1. Condition of subject—stout, emaciated, decomposed etc.	2. Wounds—position, size, character	3. Bruises—position, size and nature	4. Marks of ligature on neck, dissection etc.

II. CRANIUM AND SPINAL CANAL	1. Scalp: Skull and vertebrae	2. Membrane	3. Brain and spinal cord (The spinal canal need not be examined unless any indication of disease or injury exists)

III. THORAX	1. Walls, ribs and cartilages	2. Pleurae	3. Larynx and trachea	Right lung	Left lung	Pericardium	Heart	Vessels

IV. ABDOMEN	1. Walls	2. Peritoneum	3. Mouth, pharynx and esophagus	4. Stomach and its contents	5. Small intestine and its contents	6. Large intestine and its contents
	7. Liver	8. Spleen	9. Kidneys	10. Bladder	11. Organs of generation, external and internal	

MUSCLES, BONES AND JOINTS	1. Injury	2. Disease or deformity	3. Fracture	4. Dislocation

MORE DETAILED DESCRIPTION OF INJURY OR DISEASE	
	OPINION OF THE MEDICAL OFFICER AS TO THE CAUSE OF DEATH	REMARKS BY CIVIL SURGEON
	N.B. In the case of wounded note whether there is any indication of the wounds being homicidal, sucidal or otherwise	
	Assistant Surgeon of...	*Civil Surgeon of..*
		The day of 20

West Bengal Form No. 5372

POSTMORTEM REPORT

(P.R.B. Form No. 55 - Vide Rule 284)

STATION ....

..............day of..........20.....

Name, sex, age and caste	Whence brought: Village and Thana	Name of Constable by whom brought and names of relatives accompanying	Date and hour of Despatch	Date and hour of Arrival at dead-house	Date and hour of Examination	Information furnished by Police	By whom identified before the Medical Officer

N. B. - Observe the state of all the organs and when no disease or inury is found write "Healthy"

I. EXTERNAL APPEARANCE

1. Condition of subject—stout, emaciated, decomposed etc.	2. Wounds—position, size, character	3. Bruises—position, size and nature	4. Marks of ligature on neck, dissection etc.

II. CRANIUM AND SPINAL CANAL

1. Scalp: Skull and vertebrae	2. Membrane	3. Brain and spinal cord (The spinal canal need not be examined unless any indication of disease or injury exists)

III. THORAX

1. Walls, ribs and cartilages	2. Pleurae	3. Larynx and trachea	Right lung	Left lung	Pericardium	Heart	Vessels

IV. ABDOMEN

1. Walls	2. Peritoneum	3. Mouth, pharynx and esophagus	4. Stomach and its contents	5. Small intestine and its contents	6. Large intestine and its contents

7. Liver	8. Spleen	9. Kidneys	10. Bladder	11. Organs of generation, external and internal

MUSCLES, BONES AND JOINTS

1. Injury	2. Disease or deformity	3. Fracture	4. Dislocation

MORE DETAILED DESCRIPTION OF INJURY OR DISEASE

OPINION OF THE MEDICAL OFFICER AS TO THE CAUSE OF DEATH	REMARKS BY CIVIL SURGEON
N.B. In the case of wounded note whether there is any indication of the wounds being homicidal, sucidal or otherwise *Assistant Surgeon of*..	*Civil Surgeon of*.. *The* *day of* *20*

West Bengal Form No. 5372

POSTMORTEM REPORT

(P.R.B. Form No. 55 - Vide Rule 284)

STATION ....

...............day of...........20.....

Name, sex, age and caste	Whence brought: Village and Thana	Name of Constable by whom brought and names of relatives accompanying	Date and hour of			Information furnished by Police	By whom identified before the Medical Officer
			Despatch	Arrival at dead-house	Examination		

N. B. - Observe the state of all the organs and when no disease or inury is found write "Healthy"

I. EXTERNAL APPEARANCE	1. Condition of subject—stout, emaciated, decomposed etc.	2. Wounds—position, size, character	3. Bruises—position, size and nature	4. Marks of ligature on neck, dissection etc.

II. CRANIUM AND SPINAL CANAL	1. Scalp: Skull and vertebrae	2. Membrane	3. Brain and spinal cord (The spinal canal need not be examined unless any indication of disease or injury exists)

III. THORAX	1. Walls, ribs and cartilages	2. Pleurae	3. Larynx and trachea	Right lung	Left lung	Pericardium	Heart	Vessels

IV. ABDOMEN	1. Walls	2. Peritoneum	3. Mouth, pharynx and esophagus	4. Stomach and its contents	5. Small intestine and its contents	6. Large intestine and its contents

IV. ABDOMEN	7. Liver	8. Spleen	9. Kidneys	10. Bladder	11. Organs of generation, external and internal

MUSCLES, BONES AND JOINTS	1. Injury	2. Disease or deformity	3. Fracture	4. Dislocation

MORE DETAILED DESCRIPTION OF INJURY OR DISEASE	

OPINION OF THE MEDICAL OFFICER AS TO THE CAUSE OF DEATH	REMARKS BY CIVIL SURGEON
N.B. In the case of wounded note whether there is any indication of the wounds being homicidal, sucidal or otherwise *Assistant Surgeon of*..	*Civil Surgeon of*.. *The* *day of* *20*

West Bengal Form No. 5372

POSTMORTEM REPORT

(P.R.B. Form No. 55 - Vide Rule 284)

STATION ....

..............day of..........20.....

	Name, sex, age and caste	Whence brought: Village and Thana	Name of Constable by whom brought and names of relatives accompanying	Date and hour of			Information furnished by Police	By whom identified before the Medical Officer
				Despatch	Arrival at dead-house	Examination		

N. B. - Observe the state of all the organs and when no disease or inury is found write "Healthy"

I. EXTERNAL APPEARANCE	1. Condition of subject—stout, emaciated, decomposed etc.	2. Wounds—position, size, character	3. Bruises—position, size and nature	4. Marks of ligature on neck, dissection etc.

II. CRANIUM AND SPINAL CANAL	1. Scalp: Skull and vertebrae	2. Membrane	3. Brain and spinal cord (The spinal canal need not be examined unless any indication of disease or injury exists)

III. THORAX	1. Walls, ribs and cartilages	2. Pleurae	3. Larynx and trachea	Right lung	Left lung	Pericardium	Heart	Vessels

IV. ABDOMEN	1. Walls	2. Peritoneum	3. Mouth, pharynx and esophagus	4. Stomach and its contents	5. Small intestine and its contents	6. Large intestine and its contents
	7. Liver	8. Spleen	9. Kidneys	10. Bladder	11. Organs of generation, external and internal	

MUSCLES, BONES AND JOINTS	1. Injury	2. Disease or deformity	3. Fracture	4. Dislocation

MORE DETAILED DESCRIPTION OF INJURY OR DISEASE	

	OPINION OF THE MEDICAL OFFICER AS TO THE CAUSE OF DEATH	REMARKS BY CIVIL SURGEON
	N.B. In the case of wounded note whether there is any indication of the wounds being homicidal, sucidal or otherwise	
	Assistant Surgeon of..	*Civil Surgeon of*..
		The *day of* *20*

West Bengal Form No. 5372

POSTMORTEM REPORT

(P.R.B. Form No. 55 - Vide Rule 284)

STATION ....

..............day of..........20.....

	Name, sex, age and caste	Whence brought: Village and Thana	Name of Constable by whom brought and names of relatives accompanying	Date and hour of			Information furnished by Police	By whom identified before the Medical Officer
				Despatch	Arrival at dead-house	Examination		

N. B. - Observe the state of all the organs and when no disease or inury is found write "Healthy"

I. EXTERNAL APPEARANCE	1. Condition of subject—stout, emaciated, decomposed etc.	2. Wounds—position, size, character	3. Bruises—position, size and nature	4. Marks of ligature on neck, dissection etc.

II. CRANIUM AND SPINAL CANAL	1. Scalp: Skull and vertebrae	2. Membrane	3. Brain and spinal cord (The spinal canal need not be examined unless any indication of disease or injury exists)

III. THORAX	1. Walls, ribs and cartilages	2. Pleurae	3. Larynx and trachea	Right lung	Left lung	Pericardium	Heart	Vessels

IV. ABDOMEN	1. Walls	2. Peritoneum	3. Mouth, pharynx and esophagus	4. Stomach and its contents	5. Small intestine and its contents	6. Large intestine and its contents

IV. ABDOMEN	7. Liver	8. Spleen	9. Kidneys	10. Bladder	11. Organs of generation, external and internal

MUSCLES, BONES AND JOINTS	1. Injury	2. Disease or deformity	3. Fracture	4. Dislocation

MORE DETAILED DESCRIPTION OF INJURY OR DISEASE	

OPINION OF THE MEDICAL OFFICER AS TO THE CAUSE OF DEATH	REMARKS BY CIVIL SURGEON
N.B. In the case of wounded note whether there is any indication of the wounds being homicidal, sucidal or otherwise	
Assistant Surgeon of..	*Civil Surgeon of*..
	The *day of* *20*

West Bengal Form No. 5372

POSTMORTEM REPORT

(P.R.B. Form No. 55 - Vide Rule 284)

STATION ....

...............day of...........20.....

Name, sex, age and caste	Whence brought: Village and Thana	Name of Constable by whom brought and names of relatives accompanying	Date and hour of			Information furnished by Police	By whom identified before the Medical Officer
			Despatch	Arrival at dead-house	Examination		

N. B. - Observe the state of all the organs and when no disease or inury is found write "Healthy"

I. EXTERNAL APPEARANCE	1. Condition of subject—stout, emaciated, decomposed etc.	2. Wounds—position, size, character	3. Bruises—position, size and nature	4. Marks of ligature on neck, dissection etc.

II. CRANIUM AND SPINAL CANAL	1. Scalp: Skull and vertebrae	2. Membrane	3. Brain and spinal cord (The spinal canal need not be examined unless any indication of disease or injury exists)

III. THORAX	1. Walls, ribs and cartilages	2. Pleurae	3. Larynx and trachea	Right lung	Left lung	Pericardium	Heart	Vessels

IV. ABDOMEN	1. Walls	2. Peritoneum	3. Mouth, pharynx and esophagus	4. Stomach and its contents	5. Small intestine and its contents	6. Large intestine and its contents

IV. ABDOMEN	7. Liver	8. Spleen	9. Kidneys	10. Bladder	11. Organs of generation, external and internal

MUSCLES, BONES AND JOINTS	1. Injury	2. Disease or deformity	3. Fracture	4. Dislocation

MORE DETAILED DESCRIPTION OF INJURY OR DISEASE	

OPINION OF THE MEDICAL OFFICER AS TO THE CAUSE OF DEATH	REMARKS BY CIVIL SURGEON
N.B. In the case of wounded note whether there is any indication of the wounds being homicidal, sucidal or otherwise	
Assistant Surgeon of..	*Civil Surgeon of*..
	The *day of* *20*

West Bengal Form No. 5372

POSTMORTEM REPORT

(P.R.B. Form No. 55 - Vide Rule 284)

STATION ....

..............day of..........20.....

	Name, sex, age and caste	Whence brought: Village and Thana	Name of Constable by whom brought and names of relatives accompanying	Date and hour of			Information furnished by Police	By whom identified before the Medical Officer
				Despatch	Arrival at dead-house	Examination		

N. B. - Observe the state of all the organs and when no disease or inury is found write "Healthy"

I. EXTERNAL APPEARANCE	1. Condition of subject—stout, emaciated, decomposed etc.	2. Wounds—position, size, character	3. Bruises—position, size and nature	4. Marks of ligature on neck, dissection etc.

II. CRANIUM AND SPINAL CANAL	1. Scalp: Skull and vertebrae	2. Membrane	3. Brain and spinal cord (The spinal canal need not be examined unless any indication of disease or injury exists)

III. THORAX	1. Walls, ribs and cartilages	2. Pleurae	3. Larynx and trachea	Right lung	Left lung	Pericardium	Heart	Vessels

IV. ABDOMEN	1. Walls	2. Peritoneum	3. Mouth, pharynx and esophagus	4. Stomach and its contents	5. Small intestine and its contents	6. Large intestine and its contents
	7. Liver	8. Spleen	9. Kidneys	10. Bladder	11. Organs of generation, external and internal	

MUSCLES, BONES AND JOINTS	1. Injury	2. Disease or deformity	3. Fracture	4. Dislocation

MORE DETAILED DESCRIPTION OF INJURY OR DISEASE	

OPINION OF THE MEDICAL OFFICER AS TO THE CAUSE OF DEATH	REMARKS BY CIVIL SURGEON
N.B. In the case of wounded note whether there is any indication of the wounds being homicidal, sucidal or otherwise	
Assistant Surgeon of..	*Civil Surgeon of*..
	The *day of* *20*

West Bengal Form No. 5372

POSTMORTEM REPORT

(P.R.B. Form No. 55 - Vide Rule 284)

STATION ....

...............day of...........20.....

Name, sex, age and caste	Whence brought: Village and Thana	Name of Constable by whom brought and names of relatives accompanying	Date and hour of			Information furnished by Police	By whom identified before the Medical Officer
			Despatch	Arrival at dead-house	Examination		

N. B. - Observe the state of all the organs and when no disease or inury is found write "Healthy"

I. EXTERNAL APPEARANCE

1. Condition of subject—stout, emaciated, decomposed etc.	2. Wounds—position, size, character	3. Bruises—position, size and nature	4. Marks of ligature on neck, dissection etc.

II. CRANIUM AND SPINAL CANAL

1. Scalp: Skull and vertebrae	2. Membrane	3. Brain and spinal cord (The spinal canal need not be examined unless any indication of disease or injury exists)

III. THORAX

1. Walls, ribs and cartilages	2. Pleurae	3. Larynx and trachea	Right lung	Left lung	Pericardium	Heart	Vessels

IV. ABDOMEN

1. Walls	2. Peritoneum	3. Mouth, pharynx and esophagus	4. Stomach and its contents	5. Small intestine and its contents	6. Large intestine and its contents

7. Liver	8. Spleen	9. Kidneys	10. Bladder	11. Organs of generation, external and internal

MUSCLES, BONES AND JOINTS

1. Injury	2. Disease or deformity	3. Fracture	4. Dislocation

MORE DETAILED DESCRIPTION OF INJURY OR DISEASE

OPINION OF THE MEDICAL OFFICER AS TO THE CAUSE OF DEATH	REMARKS BY CIVIL SURGEON
N.B. In the case of wounded note whether there is any indication of the wounds being homicidal, sucidal or otherwise	
Assistant Surgeon of..	*Civil Surgeon of*..
	The *day of* *20*

West Bengal Form No. 5372

POSTMORTEM REPORT

(P.R.B. Form No. 55 - Vide Rule 284)

STATION ....

..............day of..........20.....

Name, sex, age and caste	Whence brought: Village and Thana	Name of Constable by whom brought and names of relatives accompanying	Date and hour of Despatch	Date and hour of Arrival at dead-house	Date and hour of Examination	Information furnished by Police	By whom identified before the Medical Officer

N. B. - Observe the state of all the organs and when no disease or inury is found write "Healthy"

I. EXTERNAL APPEARANCE

1. Condition of subject—stout, emaciated, decomposed etc.	2. Wounds—position, size, character	3. Bruises—position, size and nature	4. Marks of ligature on neck, dissection etc.

II. CRANIUM AND SPINAL CANAL

1. Scalp: Skull and vertebrae	2. Membrane	3. Brain and spinal cord (The spinal canal need not be examined unless any indication of disease or injury exists)

III. THORAX

1. Walls, ribs and cartilages	2. Pleurae	3. Larynx and trachea	Right lung	Left lung	Pericardium	Heart	Vessels

IV. ABDOMEN

1. Walls	2. Peritoneum	3. Mouth, pharynx and esophagus	4. Stomach and its contents	5. Small intestine and its contents	6. Large intestine and its contents

7. Liver	8. Spleen	9. Kidneys	10. Bladder	11. Organs of generation, external and internal

MUSCLES, BONES AND JOINTS

1. Injury	2. Disease or deformity	3. Fracture	4. Dislocation

MORE DETAILED DESCRIPTION OF INJURY OR DISEASE

OPINION OF THE MEDICAL OFFICER AS TO THE CAUSE OF DEATH	REMARKS BY CIVIL SURGEON
N.B. In the case of wounded note whether there is any indication of the wounds being homicidal, sucidal or otherwise *Assistant Surgeon of*..	*Civil Surgeon of*.. *The* *day of* *20*

West Bengal Form No. 5372

POSTMORTEM REPORT

(P.R.B. Form No. 55 - Vide Rule 284)

STATION ....

..............day of..........20.....

Name, sex, age and caste	Whence brought: Village and Thana	Name of Constable by whom brought and names of relatives accompanying	Date and hour of			Information furnished by Police	By whom identified before the Medical Officer
			Despatch	Arrival at dead-house	Examination		

N. B. - Observe the state of all the organs and when no disease or inury is found write "Healthy"

I. EXTERNAL APPEARANCE

1. Condition of subject—stout, emaciated, decomposed etc.	2. Wounds—position, size, character	3. Bruises—position, size and nature	4. Marks of ligature on neck, dissection etc.

II. CRANIUM AND SPINAL CANAL

1. Scalp: Skull and vertebrae	2. Membrane	3. Brain and spinal cord (The spinal canal need not be examined unless any indication of disease or injury exists)

III. THORAX

1. Walls, ribs and cartilages	2. Pleurae	3. Larynx and trachea	Right lung	Left lung	Pericardium	Heart	Vessels

IV. ABDOMEN

1. Walls	2. Peritoneum	3. Mouth, pharynx and esophagus	4. Stomach and its contents	5. Small intestine and its contents	6. Large intestine and its contents

7. Liver	8. Spleen	9. Kidneys	10. Bladder	11. Organs of generation, external and internal

MUSCLES, BONES AND JOINTS

1. Injury	2. Disease or deformity	3. Fracture	4. Dislocation

MORE DETAILED DESCRIPTION OF INJURY OR DISEASE

OPINION OF THE MEDICAL OFFICER AS TO THE CAUSE OF DEATH	REMARKS BY CIVIL SURGEON
N.B. In the case of wounded note whether there is any indication of the wounds being homicidal, sucidal or otherwise *Assistant Surgeon of*..	*Civil Surgeon of*.. *The* *day of* *20*